AF724984

Praise for Robert J. Shearer

"Shearer has documented his journey as a cancer caregiver. *We Were Better Together* is a true labor of love, very inspiring– an outstanding tribute to his wife Melissa that is sure to help countless cancer patients along their journey."

—Cliff Megerian, MD, health system CEO and ENT surgeon

"*We Were Better Together* is a beautifully written book and companion for patients and their loved ones living in an unimaginable situation. Every individual travels their own unique journey with many ups and downs, and the anguishes and fears and hopes are shared by family and close friends. The author advances a unique and valuable guide to embrace and succeed in this difficult pathway with excellent advice both spiritually and scientifically. This book is essential reading for patients and family."

—Jeffrey Miller, MD, pulmonologist and critical care physician

"Although ostensibly about one couple's eight-year cancer battle, Shearer has packed this comprehensive guidebook with the kind of advice every couple can use to deepen their bonds and work through difficulties. His choice of experts is impressive. These leaders in their fields impart knowledge in clear, easily understandable language. Bravo!"

—Dean Borth, MD, F.A.C.S. Board-certified general surgeon

"*We Were Better Together* influenced me deeply. Bob's love for his wife manifests as love for all of us. It is practical, insightful, real and provides hope to anyone who is touched by cancer personally, through a loved one or as a caregiver. You must read it."

—Francoise Adan, MD, chief leader of a nationally-recognized integrative health program and psychiatrist, immediate past Board Chair of the Academic Consortium of Integrative Medicine and Health

We Were Better Together

ROBERT J. SHEARER
with Karen Bussen

Copyright © 2024 by Robert J. Shearer

All rights reserved.

No part of this book may be reproduced in any form or by any electronic or mechanical means, including information storage and retrieval systems, without written permission from the author, except for the use of brief quotations in a book review.

ISBN: 978-1-956955-99-6 (ebook)

ISBN: 978-1-956955-98-9 (paperback)

ISBN: 978-1-964377-04-9 (hardcover)

Cover design by One Graphica

Interior design layout by Noble Thread Designs

Although the publisher and the author have made every effort to ensure that the information in this book was correct at press time, and while this publication is designed to provide accurate information in regard to the covered subject matter, the publisher and the author assume no responsibility for errors, inaccuracies, omissions, or any other inconsistencies herein and hereby disclaim any liability to any party for any loss, damage, or disruption caused by errors or omissions, whether such errors or omissions result from negligence, accident, or any other cause.

The publisher and the author are not medical professionals and the content of this book is for informational purposes only. The information presented is the author's opinion and does not constitute any health or medical advice. It is not intended to diagnose, treat, cure or prevent any condition is a disease, and readers should not use this book as a substitute for consultations with a licensed practitioner. Readers accept the risk that results may differ for each individual, and the publisher and author make no representations or guarantees of success, including as it relates to the opinions of featured experts.

Likewise, this book is not intended to be a source of financial or legal advice. Making adjustments to a financial strategy or plan should only be undertaken after consulting with a professional.

To the maximum extent permitted by law, the publisher and the author disclaim any and all liability in the event any information, commentary, analysis, opinions, advice and/or recommendations contained in this book prove to be inaccurate, incomplete or unreliable, or result in any investment or other losses.

This book is dedicated to my beautiful wife, Melissa, but also to our families, in thanks for the support they always offered us during our life together, and for the loving care they showed me after I lost her.

Table of Contents

FOREWORD

I met Bob Shearer more than 35 years ago, in a business relationship that quickly evolved into a friendship that grew deeper over time. In 2015, we became bound by a common thread after my wife, Connie, and Bob's wife, Melissa, were both diagnosed with cancer within a few months of each other. In other words, we became what I refer to as "cancer cousins."

One thing Bob and I both discovered is that this journey, while difficult, can result in a beautiful bond and a deepening of love with your partner that is greater than you can ever imagine. All of those lessons are clearly evident in this book, which closely resembles the path I traveled for six years.

A cancer diagnosis is an extraordinary moment that changes the course of people's lives. It is a time when the ground shifts beneath our feet, when we find ourselves grappling with a whirlwind of emotions and uncertainties.

We Were Better Together: Navigating Cancer as a Couple plumbs the depths of the human spirit, acknowledging the fear and grief that accompany a cancer diagnosis. At the same time, it offers tools for cultivating resilience, creating meaning amidst adversity and nurturing the strength to push on and find hope.

It empowers caregivers and patients to become active participants at every waypoint, offering them advice on understanding treatment options, managing side effects and advocating for their needs within the healthcare system. It is a tribute to the courage and determination that resides within each of us.

Within these pages, you will discover a wealth of knowledge and insights that offer solace and practical advice. While Bob's inspiration for this book came from his love for Melissa—as evidenced by his letters to her, which accompany every chapter—he has also skillfully woven together the varied expertise of medical professionals, clergy, therapists and others to create a guide that embraces both the medical and human aspects of this transformative experience.

As a result, readers don't have to start at square one in their cancer journeys. Bob has done much of the legwork by interviewing many individuals who play a part in the critical support systems that can help us remain centered and strong. The advice is presented in a practical, orderly manner, covering both the emotional and logistical journey. I can tell you from personal experience that as you read, you will feel as if Bob is reading your mind.

The learning curve for dealing with cancer is steep and daunting. In the face of such profound challenges—and the accompanying stress, fear, anger and depression—we seek guidance, understanding and hope. This book is both a lifeline and a roadmap of sorts, devoted to navigating the complexities of all stages of cancer and its treatment. By writing it, Bob has cast a beacon of light to guide readers through the storm.

This is the book I wish I had read when Connie was diagnosed. I am grateful for Bob's passion in creating it, so that those who come after us can go forth with greater perspective and vision.

May this book be your trusted companion and provide you comfort, guidance and inspiration. May it empower you to take control of the process, to make informed decisions and embrace the love and fullness of life, even during great difficulties.

And may it remind you that no matter the treatment or outcome, you are never alone. There is a vast community of individuals, caregivers and healthcare professionals who stand beside you, ready to offer support and compassion.

Neil Waxman
Pepper Pike, Ohio

HOW TO USE THIS BOOK

A Note from the Author

We Were Better Together: Navigating Cancer as a Couple is centered on a cancer journey, because that's been my experience. My wife Melissa and I fought her disease together for eight years. While the book is geared toward partners who are navigating illness together, it's also intended as a resource for anyone in a couple or family dealing with a serious health issue.

I've written this guide because frankly, I wish I'd had something like it when Melissa and I were thrown into our sudden and years-long relationship with cancer. The book is the story of our love and our journey, and I've framed it through letters I wrote to Melissa after her death. I'm making these letters public, because I want others to understand how unique each couple's approach can be as they chart their own course.

Throughout this book, and as Melissa's husband and primary caregiver, I'll share the approach, thinking and routines we used to face our struggles as well as our victories along the way. Our tips and suggestions will be summarized in the Practical Advice section of each chapter.

I've also asked some wonderful experts to add perspectives and advice wherever I thought it might be helpful. Below is a little about each of them:

- Theodoros (Ted) Teknos, MD, President of an internationally recognized cancer center and head and neck surgical oncologist
- Santosh Rao, MD, Medical Director of a nationally recognized integrative oncology program and medical oncologist, President of the Society for Integrative Oncology
- J. Cameron Muir, MD, palliative care physician and Chief Innovation Officer, National Partnership for Healthcare and Hospice Innovation
- Alise G. Bartley, PhD, LMHC-S, LMFT-S, IMFT-S, LPCC-S, AAMFT clinical supervisor, AAMFT clinical fellow
- Reverend Terence Keehan (Father Terry), pastor, Holy Family Catholic Community
- Michael Milward, CEO, California Hospice Network and strategic advisor, National Partnership for Healthcare and Hospice Innovation
- Kelly Farrell-Emley, doctor of chiropractic and nutritional wellness expert
- Fran Wesley, AAI insurance expert and Vice President, Assured Partners
- Andrew Krause, veteran estate planning attorney
- Cheryl Agronavich, registered nurse and women's health expert
- Bob Kaleal, sports therapist and personal trainer
- Karen Bussen, former CEO of the end-of-life planning platform Farewelling and internationally known event expert

In each chapter's Help from the Experts section (among other places), you'll find their wisdom and guidance in the form of quotes, exercises, dialogues and essays—on everything from getting the initial diagnosis, dealing with communication, treatment, remission and transitioning through success (or the alternative).

Even so, please do note that I'm neither a medical professional nor a therapist. When it comes to science, care options and selecting specific treatment methods, absolutely do talk with your own team and seek out the resources that will best suit your needs.

With all this said, whether you are a patient, family member or caregiver and wherever you are in your personal health journey, know that you are most welcome here. I hope this book can provide you some comfort and guidance.

Robert J. Shearer

Chapter 1
BEFORE AND AFTER

My sweet Melissa,

Do you remember the first time I told you I loved you? We were sitting by the pond in the woods behind my house. That house became our first home together.

I never wanted to write this letter, nor any of the letters in this book.

Instead, I would much rather keep telling you everything over dinner in our favorite restaurant or talking softly to you in our bed at the end of the day, like always. I'd rather write you notes and attach them to small, surprise gifts to delight you and make your eyes light up with happiness. I'd rather hold your hands in mine and let you know every day how precious you are to me.

I can't do that now, because you've flown away (I still have trouble saying you've died). Yet there is so much I want to share with you, so much we still wanted to do. I'm writing this book to tell our story—not only to honor the bold and brilliant woman I met at a horse show in Adrian, Michigan in 1983, and with whom I spent more than 30 of the happiest years of my life—but hopefully also to shine some light for others navigating the same path we started traveling after your diagnosis in 2014.

Why? Because when we were thrown into the chaos of this experience, we struggled to understand the research, find the right resources and process all the options. We were lost. I know that after all we went through, and just as you always did in everything you took on, that you would've wanted me to tell our story to help as many people as possible.

Both of us would've been so grateful for some clear advice and practical guidance on what to ask, what to expect, where to turn and what to do at the beginning of our struggles. So that's where I'll start here, my darling. I hope to do you proud.

With all my love,

Bob

PRACTICAL ADVICE

With cancer, there is always a road that leads to the moment when your life changes, and it often feels like a heavy fog barreling in just when you most need clarity. In the "before" times with Melissa, our life was filled with the shared work we loved for many years at our company, Shearer Foods, which we sold about two years before Melissa was diagnosed.

We were focused on our witty friends and close family, our horses and dogs, our three homes in wonderful communities. We had an almost whimsical sense of liberty that only child-free couples who marry a bit later in life can enjoy. We had purpose and faith. We tried to give back whenever we could, and I can honestly say, we savored every moment and were always thankful.

Our story of illness began unexpectedly, as is often the case with cancer, when Melissa experienced a series of alarming symptoms while we were at our home in Florida. We knew we might be facing something serious when Melissa's primary care doctor told us we needed to get more testing "right away." There was an urgency in her voice, so we flew back to our home base in Ohio, strategizing like the entrepreneurs we were, to get ahead of the challenge and decide how to deal with whatever was coming. After about two weeks of appointments and blood work, we officially got the news.

The "after" began one morning when we found ourselves in the oncologist's office at University Hospitals Seidman Cancer Center in Cleveland, watching the doctor's mouth move yet not being able to comprehend the enormity of the words. All at once, everything had changed. We were in uncharted territory. Neither of us had ever been seriously ill, and we were, like a lot of healthy people, unprepared.

Two words—"uterine cancer"—sent us into a battle that no couple wants to fight, one that can start and end in so many different ways. For me, the immediate and urgent objective was to act aggressively to remove whatever was causing the problem—to wait not a single moment longer than was necessary and to meet the situation head-on.

Melissa and I talked it through before making a plan of attack that we approached largely like businesspeople with a crisis to solve. It was a campaign that we were winning daily for almost eight years.

Because communication and planning helped us so much at our first waypoint while navigating cancer, I wanted to fill this chapter with some practical guidance that might help if you and your partner have received a diagnosis and are at the beginning of your "after" timeline.

When Something Isn't Right

In my experience as a caregiver, and from what I've gleaned talking to close friends who've been through cancer as well, there's never a time when you're more rational and hopeful than in the very beginning, before the full diagnosis. You know something is wrong, but there are still a range of possible outcomes. You're still new to the process, so while you'll inevitably feel nervous or worried, you can use the early days pre- or post-diagnosis to strategize and talk as a couple about how to approach next steps. Of course, every couple needs to make their own decisions, but the important thing is to discuss your best strategy. For us, it all came down to one principle that anchored us: determined optimism.

In other words, we decided we would do our best to put fear aside and focus on positivity and a proactive approach. We would tackle the situation like we would have tackled a serious threat to our business, which had been such an important part of our lives. We would break down the problem and the process and refuse to give up. In the next chapter, we'll talk through jumping into treatment, but let's start here: with how to align your mindset and communicate with your partner to set yourselves up for a better experience.

Post-Diagnosis: Make Space and Time to Talk to Your Partner

If you're reading this book, you might have already received a scary diagnosis. This is such a difficult moment, as immediately following this type of news, you'll likely feel not just genuinely frightened, but shocked, confused, upset and completely overwhelmed. This is totally normal. In Chapter Two, we'll explore techniques for communicating with your partner in more depth through conversation with an expert—but for now, here are my tips on things that worked for Melissa and me as we stepped into this new landscape to get you started.

It's okay to cry, be angry and let whatever feelings you're experiencing surface. This applies throughout the whole course of an illness, but even more so at the beginning. Since the early stages of a cancer journey can seem shameful or even taboo, support each other openly and set the tone for honest and mutual communication.

Don't minimize the difficult emotions, the exhaustion, the changes in behaviors. Allow room for this transition. Most of all, listen to your partner—*really* listen. Sometimes an answer or solution to a voiced problem is not what's actually needed, so resist giving "good advice" or "pep talks" to motivate or push your partner. Instead, embrace the art of listening, because simply being heard can be restorative. Focus on support and comfort first before beginning to address the important questions that will shape your way going forward.

While we were seeing doctors and awaiting test results, Melissa and I suspected something was wrong, but we were still in hopeful denial somewhat. Once the diagnosis made everything real, I remember telling Melissa not to worry, that I would be there with her every step of the way and that we'd get through it all together. I realized I'd have to take on the caregiver role, which was a serious commitment. In light of all this, we knew there was no turning back. We had to move full steam ahead with treatment, and I would do everything I could to provide Melissa the best care and comfort possible, physically and mentally.

Although I knew she didn't like any kind of medical procedure, Melissa rarely mentioned her fear, though because I knew her so well, I knew she was afraid. I thought the treatments (needles and such) would bother her more than the disease itself, but she never wavered. More than once, she told me that she actually liked getting chemo because she felt it was having a positive effect on her health. She never questioned the process. She just asked, "When do we start?"

As partners, I remember there was a period of quietness in our communication after the diagnosis. In retrospect, I suppose we were doing our initial processing. When that passed, we came together for conversation and planning.

You will need time and space to accept your new reality as a couple and as individuals, but if I could give one piece of advice, I'd say that it is essential to tell your partner—and more importantly, to show them—that you'll be by their side, no matter what.

To Share or Not to Share

How do you decide whether to let others know what's going on and in how much detail? This can be a difficult decision for some couples, but for Melissa and me, it was straightforward: She wanted to tell no one.

I understood her argument. She was a vibrant woman who loved to be there for others. She was the first person her friends called when they needed good advice about almost anything. She loved life, dinner parties, travel and laughter, and she didn't want everyone to look at her differently. Pity would have destroyed her.

I disagreed with her mainly because I knew her friends and close family would want to support her, and because I thought if it had been me, I would have wanted all the love and care I could get. But I always reminded myself that it was her story to tell, not mine.

If you do decide to tell your family, friends, and/or larger community, take time to think about the implications of it all. How often will you share updates? Are you mentally prepared to individually answer all the text messages and calls? Fortunately, there are great resources online now that can help you create updates and distribute them to a list of contacts you choose. Taking advantage of applications and sites like this can reduce the burden of being the communicator-in-chief and your partner's primary caregiver simultaneously.

Check Your Insurance—Really

We'll dive deeper into practical matters in the next chapter, but since health insurance plays such a major role in healing in the US, I strongly suggest reaching out to your insurance provider to make sure you understand what the next steps should be, whom you'll need to contact and what procedures you'll need to follow when choosing doctors, hospitals or medical centers and authorizing treatments. Since I think it's crucial to do this as soon as possible, I've included an expert conversation about insurance later in this chapter.

Start a Journal

This may seem like insignificant advice right now, but I really encourage you to buy a notebook and to record your experiences and feelings over time. In fact, it can be a wonderful exercise for both you and your partner, and may prompt deeper conversations and exchanges. I didn't start a journal early in the process, and it is one of the only things I truly regret. I would've loved to have captured some of the small moments, the jokes, the tears, the victories we shared and even the frustrations about treatment. At the end of each day, Melissa and I always made a list of three things we were grateful for, and I wish more than anything that I'd written those down so I could look through them now.

Here are a few journal prompts to inspire you, whether you are the caregiver or the patient:

How does this new reality make me feel?
How do I want to be supportive of my partner?
What do I need to do to support myself right now?

If you do start journaling, don't put pressure on yourself; just write what you feel and what comes naturally, even if it's only a few words. You'll be glad you did.

HELP FROM THE EXPERTS

In any crisis, it's important to have a foundation from which to view the experience and take comfort. For many people, a faith practice or spiritual attitude can be a cornerstone of that foundation, just as it was for Melissa and me.

We were lucky enough to have someone in the family who is a dynamic and inspirational faith leader and a true role model: Melissa's first cousin, Reverend Terence Keehan. Father Terry, as we call him, is someone who greatly influenced Melissa in her growing service to the community, and he was much more than just a religious figure. To Melissa, he was a source of wisdom, friendship and good counsel over the years.

In the conversation below, Father Terry and I talk about the power of using your spiritual framework to help you through a battle with serious illness.

ACTIVATING YOUR FAITH OR SPIRITUALITY AS A TOOL IN HEALING: A Conversation with Reverend Terence Keehan (Father Terry)

Robert J. Shearer: How can a couple use their faith to help them deal with the initial shock and fear of the unknown that comes with a cancer diagnosis?

Rev. Terence Keehan: One of the greatest honors in my work is leading couples through their marriage vows, and at a certain point in that beautiful ritual, we come to the expression "for better or worse." The older I get, I ask myself more and more in that moment, "Do they know what that means? Do they really know what 'for worse' means?" The truth is no, they don't. You never know.

There is a mystery to the commitment people make, and "worse" manifests itself in a lot of ways. "Worse" comes along and it's almost always unexpected. It's new territory. A relationship can crumble or grow closer, even in the midst of "worse." For couples who have a regular ritual or practice of faith or spirituality long before "worse" comes along, it can be true that they might have more pillars to lean on as their marriage evolves and they confront difficulties.

Also, I would like to acknowledge that there are many paths to God that many faith traditions are built on, and I encourage anyone reading this to tap into your faith traditions or spiritual wisdom particularly in moments of difficulty and crisis.

That being said, I often hear from folks who say, "I'm spiritual but not religious." And you know what? I don't think any statement can be more true: *We are all fundamentally spiritual.* In any moment of challenge, we *do* have what we need within us. We are spiritual by nature. That spirituality can come forth through the structure of religion, or through a practice a couple has together, which can be as simple as taking a walk with a greater appreciation of and attention to the beauty of creation. There is a reservoir within us, and we can dip into it at any time.

Other examples of practices include listening to meaningful music together, reading, going through old photos or reviewing some of the tools you used as a couple throughout your marriage. You might also consider a more formal program, such as a couples retreat.

RJS: Would you offer any different advice about faith or spiritual practice to the patient starting treatment as opposed to their caregiver/partner who will be there to support them? For Melissa and me, we had our own individual rituals and said our prayers together as a couple.

RTK: You know, it's really three dimensions—it's your individual prayer or practice, your rituals or beliefs as a couple and your experience with a larger community.

The majority of the time, when people have a significant level of struggle, be it through illness or another serious challenge, one of the first feelings is, you know, nobody understands what this is. I have a master's in communications, and in one class, we talked about the importance of stating the obvious. So it can be really helpful to acknowledge, "Yes, it's true, nobody knows exactly what we're going through." But that being said, could it still help to connect with others who are going through things that are at least *similar*?

As an example, Bob, you're sharing your experience in service of others by reaching out and connecting with them. That type of connection can be a real gift on both sides, and it can appear in many different ways. At our church, we've just started a group for people navigating serious illness, and we hope it will foster that exchange of experience, empathy and understanding.

RJS: What if you have feelings of guilt that you've not been attending services or not been "good enough" at your faith lately? How can you overcome those feelings and rejoin the community?

RTK: You are already a part of the community, and that doesn't change simply because of illness or setback. If you want to come back, you shouldn't stay with feelings of guilt. They are not important or helpful. We are here for you. Every single faith leader of any denomination—we are here for you, we welcome you. So just don't hesitate. Come back. The door is open.

RJS: What are some ways a couple or family can bring spirituality into their daily lives during the early, chaotic and stressful days of a cancer journey? Should they set aside a specific time each morning or evening?

RTK: I'm a big Jesuit spirituality guy. St. Ignatius of Loyola, founder of the Jesuits, a Catholic missionary community, created a really simple but profound exercise to practice every evening before you go to bed. It's called The Examen. You set aside time to reflect on your day, and you invite God to join you in your reflection, so God is reflecting with you. When you review your day, something will always catch your attention.

Observe your feelings about that something—are they fear, humor, awe, frustration? Just acknowledge what you're feeling for a moment or two. Then, give thanks to God for the day. This is a wonderful way to draw your attention to your emotions and to cultivate a closeness to God.

Another really good tool is Scripture. It may sound too easy, but just google "scripture passages about hope"—or resilience or anger or whatever you need at that moment. Read and meditate, and you'll very likely find some peace and comfort.

* * *

We'll hear more from Father Terry later in the book, but I hope this conversation will help spark meaningful discussion between you and your partner about shared faith principles and how you might use them for support in this challenging time.

Next, although it may seem a bit of a departure from our discussion about faith, I want to focus on something more earthly and practical that should ideally be addressed as soon as possible when confronting a serious illness. It's no one's favorite topic, but since health insurance is so complicated yet so integral to getting the care you need, I want to prioritize it right here in Chapter One.

To that end, I sought out expert guidance from Fran Wesley, who has been a trusted advisor to Melissa and me for years on all things insurance. As you sort through your coverage and search for all the help you need to heal, I hope you'll find some helpful advice in the conversation below.

NAVIGATING THE COMPLEXITIES OF INSURANCE BEFORE AND DURING AN ILLNESS: Valuable Advice from Fran Wesley, AAI Insurance Expert and Vice President, Assured Partners

Robert J. Shearer: Thank you so much for sharing your expertise around a subject that I think we can all agree is one of the most stressful and confusing during a health crisis: insurance. Most people don't even like to think about insurance and all of its complexities. How did you end up choosing this as a career?

Fran Wesley: Actually, it was the industry that chose me and not the other way around, but it's turned out to be a great career. After graduating from college, I went on a job interview with an insurance company, and I aced the math test. They hired me on the spot and here I am, fifty years later. Being able to help people, especially when they're planning for or going through some of life's most difficult moments, is really fulfilling for me.

RJS: Well, we have a real opportunity for you to help people here with your knowledge. Let's start at the beginning. If you're lucky enough to be able to plan in advance for health insurance, are there details you should look for in a policy that may protect you or provide extra benefits in cases of serious illness?

FW: Without a doubt. If you're lucky enough to be able to plan ahead, I always recommend choosing a plan with a high deductible, normally in the range of $3,000 to $5,000 annually, followed by 100 percent coverage when purchasing insurance.

Why? Well, first of all, when you're healthy, there are substantial savings, because a high-deductible plan is generally less expensive. Secondly, it is considerably less confusing. When you reach that deductible threshold, even though it can seem like a lot of money, everything else is 100 percent covered. You don't have to worry about the bills that arrive because your insurance carrier will pay all of the rest—100 percent.

A third advantage is if you contribute the same amount or more than your deductible into a Health Savings Account (HSA), which you're only eligible for with certain high-deductible insurance plans, you get the added benefit of being able to pay for your medical expenses with pre-tax dollars, which means you can actually break even in fewer than two years. You can also keep contributing money to your HSA year after year without paying taxes on it, letting it grow tax-free and withdrawing from it tax-free to cover future deductibles or any other high, out-of-pocket medical expenses.[1]

RJS: But should you work with an agent on this? I think a lot of people are just so overwhelmed by insurance that they honestly don't even know how to select the best plan.

FW: Yes, I strongly recommend that you purchase through an agent. Working with an agent doesn't cost you a dime, because their fees are paid by the insurance company—but when you engage a professional, you're gaining an expert who can answer questions and steer you toward the right policy.

Also, your agent is your advocate. Down the road, if you have a billing or coverage question, they are there for you. They can go to the insurance provider directly and ask, "Why are you not paying this?" That relationship can be really meaningful.

That leads to my next point: There are actually significant disadvantages to seeking insurance coverage by yourself. I'll give you an example. In my experience, people really don't understand how costs break down across different policy options when you do have a significant medical expense. As an agent, I can very easily show them the actual math with a comparison between that recommended high-deductible plan and a common 80/20 plan, where the insurance carrier pays 80 percent and you pay 20.

When I show clients that they're saving money on that high-deductible plan even when they're healthy, that's always a great exercise. But then I'll present the numbers showing that even in the event of significant medical expenses, they still don't spend more. When they see it in black and white on paper, that's when it clicks.

RJS: Can you say a bit more about how an 80/20 plan works with health insurance?

FW: Of course. If we have what we call a 100 percent policy that has a high-deductible of, say, $5,000, the client knows they have to pay the first $5,000—but that after that deductible is reached, the insurance will pay 100 percent of all other covered expenses.

With an 80/20 plan, you might have a $5,000 deductible, but once you've met that limit, any other expenses that come in are split on the 80/20 ratio. So, if your monthly medical bills for a serious illness come to $10,000, your carrier will pay $8,000 and you'll be required to pay $2,000—and generally speaking, that keeps on happening until your total out-of-pocket expenses hit some higher number than the $5,000 you'd see on a high-deductible plan with 100 percent coverage.

All of this means that the total you pay out of pocket may be much higher with an 80/20 plan than a 100 percent plan. First you have your deductible, then you have a copay for every visit and so on—

whereas when you have a 100 percent plan, you know the limits of what you'll have to pay and you're sure of your coverage beyond that amount.

And as I mentioned before, if you're really smart, you can contribute the same amount or more as your deductible to an HSA each year so you can pay for all your medical expenses with pre-tax dollars. In my own experience, I've chosen this type of plan for as long as it's been offered, and I max out my HSA annually and use that pre-tax money to pay for prescriptions and the like. It can mean significant savings, and it's easy to do.

RJS: How do you find a good agent?

FW: The best way, in my opinion, is by word of mouth. Ask someone you trust who they use, or ask your home insurance agent for a recommendation. They should be accredited, friendly and open to answering all your questions.

RJS: When it comes to insurance, what are the first steps you should take after receiving a diagnosis of an illness such as cancer? Do you call your insurance company right away? If so, whom exactly do you call?

FW: Absolutely, you should contact your insurance carrier as soon as possible. If you do have an agent, call them first. And if your coverage is through your employer, there will almost definitely be an agent.

You'll want to have a conversation with the agent to make sure you stay in-network to minimize your out-of-pocket expenses, and it's important to note that even if you buy coverage on your own, you can still work with an agent. The difference is that it may be an agent who only works for that particular carrier, whether it's UnitedHealthcare, Medical Mutual or the like. If you work with an independent agent, they will be looking across all the options to help you find the right policy, and they are not beholden to any one company. But even an exclusive agent who works only with your insurance provider can assist you after a diagnosis.

RJS: If someone hasn't worked with an agent before, how can they avoid pitfalls after getting a diagnosis?

FW: Well, once you're in a plan, if you receive a diagnosis, the options are definitely limited to what's in that plan. If your health plan comes through your employer, you don't necessarily have a lot of choice in terms of switching carriers.

If you're over 65 and have coverage outside of an employer, there is an open enrollment period that allows you to switch companies.

The important thing to note is that if you decide to change insurance providers after a diagnosis, you will have to go through "underwriting", which means they evaluate you as a candidate to decide whether to offer you coverage, which can be unlikely in certain serious or expensive situations.

RJS: Let's talk a bit more about this. If someone has insurance through work but the policy doesn't really offer the best coverage, what can they do? Can they buy another policy?

FW: Yes, but the cost is high and they will have to be underwritten by a new insurance provider. It might not be a viable option.

When employees are opting into health plans at work, they can see how much that policy is costing their employer, and those high numbers can discourage employees from looking elsewhere. They're not likely going to say, "I'm going somewhere else," because if they did, those costs would be transferred to them personally. It just doesn't make sense in most cases.

RJS: What are the questions you might want to ask when choosing an insurance policy to make sure you understand your rights and the processes you need to follow?

FW: I'm so happy you asked that, because this is very important. Here are a few to keep in mind:

- What is my deductible?
- What are my copays for visits, medications and specialists?
- What is my maximum out-of-pocket expense for the year?
- Is there a maximum amount of coverage after which my policy maxes out and I become liable for all additional expenses?
- Whom do I call when I have questions?
- If I'm unhappy, whom do I contact to appeal any decision that has been made regarding my care and the associated expenses?

RJS: When it comes to long-term illness such as cancer, what are some of the important differences between private insurance, Medicare and Medicaid?

FW: When it comes to private insurance, most is purchased through an employer as a benefit. But if you're under 65 years old and you're not employed, you'll need to purchase an individual plan. As we've already discussed, I suggest contacting an agent for guidance so you can find the right policy. That will involve a deductible, copays and other terms.

To take advantage of regular or basic Medicare, you must sign up at age 65 to avoid a penalty. This is very important, because it's a cost penalty that lasts forever, so don't skip this step when you turn 65.

Even if you're employed and currently covered under your group plan, you still need to apply for Part A of Medicare at age 65. It costs nothing, but it has to be on record. You may never use it, but you have to sign up for it.

When you're no longer under an employee group plan, you'll then want to purchase Part B, which is your doctor coverage, and Part D, your prescription coverage. The cost of this will be paid automatically out of your Social Security benefits.

After you've purchased Part B and D, you can also purchase supplemental and optional coverage through Medicare. Supplemental coverage has a lot of options, such as the 80/20 plan versus a high-deductible 100 percent plan. Even at age 65 and beyond, with Medicare supplemental plans, you have those options. Your agent can help you determine what works for you.

And then Medicaid serves people with disabilities or those who fall within a very low income range. I'm not a Medicaid expert, but more information can be found at Medicaid.gov.

RJS: Another thing that confuses people is Medicare Advantage plans. Could you just say a bit about those?

FW: Yes, these can be really misleading and confusing. They are often advertised as "zero monthly cost, zero copay, zero prescription drug cost." They sound attractive, because it seems as if they don't cost anything at all, but you must be fully aware of the disadvantages. One is that you must stay within the specified network. If you go out-of-network for anything other than an emergency, you will have exactly zero coverage.

So for example, if you're over 65 on a Medicare Advantage plan and you're traveling, you might not have an in-network option. If you become ill and/or have an accident and go to the emergency room, only the emergency room portion of the billing would be covered. For any and all follow-up care, being out-of-network, you would not be covered and would find yourself with a mountain of bills. All of the follow-up care costs would be your responsibility, unless you came back to an in-network facility and doctor.

RJS: Let's do a lightning round. What are some tips or mistakes to avoid when dealing with the healthcare system and your insurance provider in general?

FW: Here are some of my most important tips:

- First and foremost, find out who to call when you have a health issue. Connect with your agent and/or your insurance company immediately upon getting a diagnosis.
- Make sure you understand your network and any restrictions on doctors and facilities you can choose.
- With regard to prescriptions, ask your insurance provider if you can obtain the drugs you need in a less expensive generic form or even in a three-month supply from a mail-order pharmacy, which may be significantly cheaper.
- Be your own advocate, and be inquisitive in advance. With a colonoscopy, for example, going through the hospital program may cost you a couple thousand dollars. But if you go through a facility that is approved by your insurance carrier, it might save you 25 percent of that cost, so you should ask.

RJS: This has been so helpful. Is there anything else you'd like to say to encourage families to better understand and get the most from their insurance?

FW: Yes. Aside from just thinking about health insurance, I always suggest buying life insurance before there is a health crisis. Then, if the patient is the main breadwinner of their family and they have a diagnosed illness that is causing financial burden, they can contact their life insurance company, as there are benefits that start before someone dies.

People often don't realize that now, most life insurance providers offer an enhanced supplemental payment if the policy holder is deemed to be terminally ill. I know that's not the desired outcome, but if that is the reality, there is a significant benefit to having this type of coverage. A life insurance provider may advance up to 50 percent of the policy benefit before death, which can be incredibly helpful to the family. Later, they'll provide the remainder of the balance after the person has passed away. Not all insurance companies offer this, but most of the major ones do.

I always make sure that my life insurance clients know this is the case. The funds can be used for day-to-day expenses, and bills can easily pile up, so this can be a really important clause to look for. There's also no additional cost, so you don't have to upgrade into it.

These conversations are my passion:helping my clients find the details in their policies that will benefit them when they really need them. And that's what any great agent should do.

CHAPTER TAKEAWAYS:

- At the beginning of a health crisis, establishing and honoring close communication with your partner is crucial to creating a supportive and caring environment for you both—deciding important things together will strengthen your bond and streamline your process
- Identifying your pillars of strength through faith or spirituality can offer comfort and hope
- Understanding and optimizing your insurance coverage can mean better care, fewer financial woes and more freedom to make decisions
- Starting a journal can be a great source of soothing and a beautiful document to have throughout your journey

"ONCE YOU CHOOSE HOPE, ANYTHING'S POSSIBLE."

—Christopher Reeve

Chapter 2
INTO THE WOODS

Melissa, my love,

Do you remember how easy everything was for us?

That time not long after we first met, when we went on a road trip to a horse show in Florida with friends? Remember how the truck engine broke down, and we had to sit there in the trailer on bales of hay—with three horses—for something like eight hours while we waited for our friends to go to the repair shop? It felt like time just flew by when we were together, when we were talking and laughing. It was effortless.

And then when we worked together or when we built a house together—wasn't it wonderful? Not to say we never had our disagreements, but we were almost always naturally aligned in our thinking and our approach to life. Laughter, love and gratitude over all. That's how I'd describe our philosophy.

When we found out about your cancer, we knew facing it would not be as easy as spending eight hours with beautiful horses and good conversation. We knew it would not be at all like building a gorgeous new home. But we didn't expect it to be something that would bring us so much closer to one another.

We decided to confront your illness directly, and we were lucky enough to have the time and resources to organize our lives around getting you the best treatment possible.

For me, it was the way we approached it, and that started right away. Getting things in order and thinking about our process helped us to be more mentally free for all that was to come, and I'm so grateful we took just a little time to think and plan. It gave us the time and space later to deeply feel the moments we shared, even the ones that weren't so easy.

Forever yours,

Bob

PRACTICAL ADVICE

During cancer treatment, and especially at the beginning, things will sometimes seem really hectic. Managing our schedules and all the new information we're getting can become overwhelming. Before Melissa was diagnosed, we had sold our business, and I was consulting and doing advisory board work for a number of organizations. When we got the news, I quit everything to take care of her, and it was a blessing to be able to do that without financial worry.

But even so, while we were getting organized, I purposely took time to cross things off my to-do list to free up time to attend every medical appointment and meeting, and to care for my beautiful wife. Here are some things that may help you as you consider your treatment options and rearrange your life to make room for this new challenge.

Choose the Best Care For You

I know a number of families who dealt with cancer and didn't always choose the most obvious medical team for their treatment journey. As I've learned, a lot goes into deciding which doctors and facilities are right for you. Sometimes that choice is made very closely with (or even exclusively by) your insurance company. Melissa and I thought that would be one of the most overwhelming aspects of our entire experience, but in the end, we didn't have to face it all on our own. Instead, we were fortunate enough to have a close friend who advised us.

In your case, you may find that your choice seems clear, or you may have several good options in mind. In any case, here are some things to think about when choosing your treatment team:

- **Diagnosis and options.** Ask your medical providers who established the diagnosis to review all the details with you so you can understand your options, agree on the treatment plan and see the way forward. As there will be a lot of information to take in, don't be afraid to ask questions—and do take notes, as you'll definitely need to refer back to them later.

- **Reputation of your doctor and facilities.** For all the medical professionals you consider working with, read their online reviews, speak with their former patients and/or patients' families and ask questions about their philosophy and processes.

- **Distance from your home.** If you live near a major metro area, you will likely be able to choose between a well-known hospital in the heart of the city or a more local group in a suburb that is more accessible for repeated appointments, blood work and last-minute needs. Convenience can make a big difference, but consider the differences between your options and do take quality into account.

- **Other services available.** Does your prospective team offer group support, nutrition services, couples therapy, holistic additions or any other add-ons?

- **Personal rapport.** Since you'll be spending a lot of time with your doctor and their colleagues, you'll want to feel really comfortable in their presence and environment. When meeting your prospective team, be diligent, take a careful look around and trust your instincts. Even a well-known doctor with a wall full of accolades should make you feel like an individual, take the time to explain things and answer any questions you have. Ask yourself: Do you feel a solid connection of care and compassion?

- **Flexibility.** If you already have existing health or wellness providers, will your new team work with them? Melissa wanted to involve her long-time nutritionist in her treatment, because she really believed that food and supplements would be key to her recovery. Through that approach, her nutritionist was able to coordinate her diet and supplement plan with her doctors, which was a real source of comfort and support for Melissa.

- **Advocating for yourself.** What you'll need will depend on your preferences and your tolerance for more or less information and opinions. You can educate yourself by seeking credible online resources to better understand options, but do remember: sometimes too much info is just too much, and it can become unhelpful or even paralyzing.

- **Ask for a patient advocate.** Patient advocates and patient navigators are a resource that many families don't know about that can be so empowering when facing serious illness. They work through your medical center or hospital and are there to help guide you through the healthcare system, every step of the way. Your hospital should provide you with a Patient Bill of Rights, which often includes information on how to contact patient advocates and navigators. In general, these professionals can help you communicate clearly with your providers, resolve your concerns and connect you to any financial or legal services you may need, alongside other support (which is sometimes as simple as a ride home from the hospital). If you're not introduced to one or given any contact information, just tell your medical team, "We'd like to speak to a patient advocate/navigator."

- **Navigating your insurance.** If you haven't done so already, I suggest calling your insurance provider immediately and taking notes on next steps (see Chapter One for more details on this).

Think About Roles and Tasks

In a relationship, especially when one person is the patient and the other the caregiver, each person's individual needs can be very different and may change over time. In our case, I was the organizer and researcher. The more Melissa read about the available science, the more she sometimes became stressed, while I found it helpful and calming to know more. I also found it useful to confide in and ask questions of a close friend whose wife was battling pancreatic cancer, because he was farther along in the process, and I learned so much from his experiences.

Task-wise, I decided to deal with general maintenance on the house before we started treatment. That included completing some repairs, modifying a few things in our master bathroom to make Melissa more comfortable and even having the car serviced and tires changed, because I knew we'd be facing long drives (more than an hour each way) several times a week for the foreseeable future. My point here is, if there's anything you can get out of the way or off your to-do list before you dive into treatment, it may be a good idea to do so. Sometimes managing the stress of daily tasks can become excessive when you're already managing so much.

Look at Your Budget

Medical bills are one of the biggest disruptors of financial stability in the US—but when you're looking at long-term treatment for cancer, it's not just medical bills that can pile up. Loss of work for one or both partners, additional costs for childcare, transportation costs and pricey nutritional needs can also come into play.

If your funds are locked up in longer-term savings, you may want to speak to your financial institution to see what changes you can make to have more money available as needed. If you'll use a credit card for certain expenses, call your card company and see if you can negotiate your interest rate. Think about small monthly expenses you might be able to eliminate or reduce to take pressure off during an already stressful time.

What About Work?

As a caregiver, will you take time off or continue working? Will you be able to have a more flexible schedule to allow for important appointments or emergencies? It can be wise to have a conversation with your boss and/or human resources team to make sure everyone is on the same page.

As the patient, what are your options? Can you schedule treatments near the weekend so you have ample recovery time? Does your employer offer any additional benefits or services? Will they be flexible with letting you work remotely so you can take short breaks when needed or avoid the office setting when your immune system is compromised from treatment?

One important resource here is the Family and Medical Leave Act. If this law applies to the company you work for, you may be provided unpaid, job-protected time off to recover from your illness, and it can apply to both patient and/or caregiver. Check with your company's human resources team early in the process so you can understand and take advantage of the rights and benefits available to you.

Plan for Spiritual and Emotional Support and Embrace the Little Things You Love

Whatever your belief system, you may want to consider adding more support wherever you can. Melissa and I were always connected to our Catholic faith, but we weren't necessarily attending Mass every week. We decided to reprioritize doing so, and it greatly enriched our treatment experience. Whether you choose a religious community, an alternative spiritual guide, an online group, a therapist or just an objective listener, having someone to lean on can be a game-changer.

Also, remember that you may need support both as a couple and as individuals.

Even if you decide not to tell your whole community about the diagnosis and treatment, I encourage you to choose a few people to confide in to help you bear the burden of this challenge. Even the strongest and most optimistic among us needs a helping hand when confronted with something so enormous and overwhelming.

Finally, there are also many little things that can become a real anchor in a chaotic situation. Melissa found a lot of joy in continuing to do the things she loved, such as making art, watching movies on the Hallmark Channel and home improvement shows on HGTV and texting with friends and family. All these things lifted her spirits and kept her engaged and inspired. Think about what you need, and honor your needs and those of your partner.

Prepare for the Unexpected in Treatment

If you've been living a relatively "healthy" life, it can be really disconcerting when a disease or the medical treatments themselves cause a serious reaction. I remember picking Melissa up off the floor after she collapsed at home following her first chemo treatment. She had become weak and dehydrated, and I had to bring her back to the hospital for monitoring. As we learned that her treatments left her incredibly tired, we had to take that into account.

We got much better at managing her reactions once we discovered certain drugs for treating nausea and got more familiar with what to expect. The process can be very scary though, especially in the beginning when everything is new.

HELP FROM THE EXPERTS

Talking to doctors, surgeons and entire teams of medical specialists can be really daunting. How should we prepare? How many questions can we ask? How can we make the most of the limited time we have with our healthcare professionals to ensure we understand and agree with our treatment options?

The conversation below highlights advice on just that subject from one of the kindest, most personable doctors I have ever met. Although he is a renowned expert, he has such a knack for communicating clearly and putting patients and their families at ease. Dr. Teknos wasn't Melissa's doctor, but he followed her case with interest and compassion.

A ROADMAP FOR CLEAR COMMUNICATION WITH YOUR DOCTOR: Important Advice from Dr. Theodoros (Ted) Teknos, MD, President of an Internationally Recognized Cancer Center and Head and Neck Surgical Oncologist

Robert J. Shearer: Aside from training and experience, what elements should the patient and their family consider when choosing a doctor for long-term cancer treatment? Is the doctor's communication style or personality even a factor? As in, "Am I comfortable with the way this doctor communicates with me, and do I feel heard and understood?"

Dr. Ted Teknos: Yes. I think first and foremost, you need to find someone exceptionally well trained in your particular cancer. There are a lot of general oncologists who can be great for certain types of disease, and then there are those who have done fellowships that focus very specifically on one given cancer. With the speed of discovery now, finding a highly skilled doctor who is focused on your type of cancer, and who is current on all the latest research, can be critically important to your care.

Equal to that is finding someone with whom you and your loved one are comfortable. That includes feeling good about their availability, their communication style and even their personality. This is truly an intimate relationship, and understandably, cancer patients hang on every single word their oncologist says, so you want to be sure you're given the time and answers you need at each and every appointment.

An easy way to remember it is to ask yourself if they meet the criteria of "The Three A's": Are they Available? Are they Affable? And will they be an Advocate for you? The personal part is sometimes downplayed—you know, "He's a great doctor, so I'll put up with the lack of connection." But that can be a mistake. As the patient, you must insist on being comfortable, and your doctor should want that for you, too.

RJS: Yes, every time we walked into Melissa's oncologist's office, there were hugs and smiles. We chatted about his dogs, our dogs. It was a friendly relationship, and we both valued that.

So, once a patient has chosen their medical team, how can they be most prepared when communicating with their oncologist? For example, should they write down questions in advance? Should they wait until the end of an appointment to ask any outstanding questions?

DTT: Coming prepared is critically important. Writing down questions to ask before you come into an appointment helps on both sides. Because there are so many anxieties and concerns that in the whirlwind of everything going on, so many times, patients will leave and later say they forgot to ask something important.

Taking the time to prepare is great, but having a mechanism or process to follow up with your doctor if you do have more questions helps as well—a phone number or an online portal, for example. You need to have a trusting relationship and a means of communication, even outside of your official appointments.

RJS: We actually had cell phone numbers for Melissa's oncologist and for her general practitioner. I know that's not always possible, and we didn't abuse it, but it sure helped knowing we had it.

DTT: Yes—it's all about trust.

RJS: A question about the internet: Does the massive amount of medical information available in articles and on websites, both good and bad, make it easier or more difficult to have good communication with your doctor?

DTT: It makes it easier in that patients can do some of their own research, but on the other hand, there are a lot of frightening things and scams out there that aim to take advantage of people in vulnerable medical positions. You have to be wary, but the beauty of the internet is that it empowers you to learn more, and you can always ask your doctor questions.

I actually have a fascinating personal experience with this. Ten years ago or so, when genomic medicine was just coming of age, one of my patients, who had a tumor in his neck, brought me an article about one of very few companies who were starting to sequence cancer tumors.

I hadn't seen this research, but it was very interesting. My team looked into it, and it checked out. We ended up sequencing this patient's tumor, and we were surprised to see that its mutations were consistent with those that would best be treated by breast cancer drugs. If that patient hadn't found that brand new technology on the internet, we wouldn't have collectively made those decisions.

The bottom line is use common sense, but keep an open mind. We take it all on a case-by-case basis. If there is scientific proof, the short answer is that the internet is great—but there's also a lot of false information out there. Your doctor can be a sounding board and source of truth, and they should be open to looking at anything you bring in and answering your questions.

I will say this: if you do find something interesting—a study or an article, for example—if you can print out a copy and bring it with you to your appointment, that can be really helpful. Then, you just need to be open to your doctor's expertise as well. She may say, you know, "This is not the standard of care," or, "I've seen this before." But it's definitely worth bringing in, and you should never feel intimidated about doing that.

RJS: What's the key to having good communication with your oncologist?

DTT: Not to repeat myself, but it all starts with a trusting relationship. You need to feel comfortable with your oncologist. More than anything, I really think they should feel like a trusted friend, an advocate, someone who you know will listen, someone who is open to your questions.

Then it becomes extremely important to be open with them about what you're feeling—about physical symptoms, of course, but even emotions and other concerns. That builds a strong patient–doctor relationship.

Most of the responsibility for this, by the way, should fall on the doctor. Of course the patient always wants an open dialogue, but because many doctors are so pressed with the number of patients they see daily and the complexity of their work, that's where patients have to look at the time they get with their oncologist as a reflection of the type of relationship they can have.

RJS: As a doctor, what aspect of patient communication do you find most challenging, or where do you see opportunity for improvement?

DTT: I think it's always most challenging when you have to deliver difficult or bad news. That's the part that is learned with experience. Young doctors just out of training don't have that experience.

I think it's always most challenging when you have to deliver difficult or bad news. It's vitally important to put yourself in a patient's or family's position when the news is difficult. I also think oncologists must provide the patient with a sense of the status of their disease, discussing goals and timelines so patients have all the information they need, especially when they have a life-threatening illness.

Doctors must ensure they always deliver bad news in an honest, empathetic, and complete way.

RJS: Sometimes the caregiver of a patient with cancer is frustrated or wants to be more involved in the process of talking to the medical team when they're not the actual patient. Is it challenging to navigate those conversations? Do you have any advice for caregivers about communicating with their loved ones' doctors?

I ask because with our first oncologist, I never had that problem. But after he left the practice and we had a new team, I didn't feel that they considered me a participant in the process, even though for eight years, I was always there for every appointment, tuned-in and interested. I'm assuming that other caregivers could have that same issue.

DTT: Yes, caregivers are so critically important to the healing process. They must be included and welcomed into these conversations and given the authority and ability to communicate directly with the treating oncologist.

Lets face it, at the moment the diagnosis is delivered, the patient is incapable of processing it all. There are so many emotions and fears. It's overwhelming, naturally. The caregiver becomes the eyes and ears for the patient in those early moments. Then later, as treatment progresses, there are physical changes in the patient that may make remembering details difficult, so the caregiver is even more important to maintaining effective communication as well as the patient's healing and overall experience. A caregiver should feel empowered to speak for and with the patient, and many times, doctors will ask the caregivers to bring in tape recorders to get the conversations so they can be processed later. This happens quite a lot now, and it's great.

RJS: As a doctor with so many different types of patients and their families, do you find that you need to deliver news, results or even opinions in different ways depending on who's receiving the info?

DTT: I think that's where a doctor's emotional intelligence comes to the fore. You develop this personal approach as you get to know patients and their families, their children, even their social situation. How you deliver information, news and challenges all depends on those relationships and what support they have. The ability to read social cues and pick up on family and patient-caregiver reactions molds how you discuss things with patients and their loved ones.

RJS: Following up on that, should patients tell their doctor *how* they like to receive news? As in preferring a give-it-to-me-straight approach versus something more nuanced?

DTT: That's a great way to phrase it: "As we develop our physician–patient relationship, how would you like to approach exchanging information? Would you prefer me to be more glass-half-full, or is it better for you if I'm as honest and forthright, but caring as I can be?" I find that most people want honest, straightforward, but kind communication, even if they are naturally optimistic. They want to know, "Where am I? What are my options? What are the chances I'll live another six months, a year, five years?"

RJS: Anything else you'd like to share about creating a strong, open channel of communication between doctors and patients to improve the overall care experience?

DTT: The most important thing is to find someone you're comfortable with—someone who is basically going to be a member of your family. I approach my patient interactions from the standpoint of wanting to become very, very close and, if possible, friends. It's an incredible privilege to take care of patients during their cancer journeys, and they have to feel likewise.

A simple question may also help you determine how confident you should be in your chosen oncologist, that being, "Would you have any objections to me getting a second opinion at some point during my treatment journey?"

If for any reason they get offended, my advice is to run the other way. That is a huge red flag. If they're confident in their credentials and their decision-making process, they should feel great about a second opinion. They should welcome it completely.

Then, I mentioned it earlier, but it bears repeating: There are many diseases that can be treated by a general oncologist—where consistent, evidence-based treatment can work really well, and you can be treated close to home, which can be a real benefit—but it's important to highlight that some diseases need complex, interdisciplinary care. You need to determine what level of expertise you need. There's evidence that for really complex cancers, patients who go to comprehensive, state-of-the art cancer care sites may have better outcomes. This especially applies to recurrent diseases and specific or metastatic cancers.

Without sounding obvious, you want the latest and greatest. What is exciting is that this is probably the most hopeful time in human history for finding cures for cancer. We can now do sequencing in a matter of hours to classify the actual genetic makeup of a tumor. With that kind of information, you can create precise personal treatments that are individual to the patient.

Leveraging genome sequencing and using artificial intelligence are all the rage, but the power of computing and genetics to personally tailor treatment really are the new Holy Grail.

Another thing we've learned from the world of genetic sequencing is that now, there are cancer therapies that activate the immune system. Immunotherapies can even help target cancers that were previously incurable, including metastatic tumors like melanoma, and the outcomes have substantially improved.

There are so many new technologies. Another exciting development is the ability to activate the immune system so it can recognize and fight a previously hidden tumor. Now, we have drugs that can "unmask" tumors so our immune systems can target them.

Beyond that, there is developing technology that allows us to take a patient's immune cells to a laboratory and modify them so they can identify a specific target on a cancer cell. Once these cells are modified, you can grow them and return them to the body. These are called chimeric antigen receptor (CAR) therapies for T-cells, also sometimes called Natural Killer (NK) cells. Through these treatments, the T-cells in our bodies become like heat-seeking missiles that can hunt tumors and eradicate them.

Our organization has one of the few facilities that can do these processes on-site. We can generate these therapies in a short window of time to literally change a person's immune system and give it the power to fight their specific cancer. The hope has never been greater.

Cancer survival rates between 1980 and 2020 have increased by 30 percent. We clearly still have a long way to go, but advances are happening at an accelerated pace.

* * *

Along with great communication strategies for talking to your healthcare team, maintaining strong communication within your relationship is equally important. You'll find more of my thoughts on prioritizing your partner in Chapter One, but for the conversation below, I wanted to bring in Dr. Alise Bartley, a dear friend who also happens to be a psychologist and a leader in her field of relationship and family counseling.

Over the years, Melissa and I have known so many people who have benefitted from Alise's work. Here, she shares some helpful advice and practices to enhance communication with your partner during a serious illness.

COMMUNICATING WITH YOUR PARTNER DURING A HEALTH CRISIS: Questions and Answers with Relationship and Family Counseling Expert Dr. Alise Bartley, AAMFT Clinical Supervisor, AAMFT Clinical Fellow

Robert J. Shearer: Melissa and I approached our communication about her cancer in the same way as we looked at our business. We specifically chose not to talk about it all the time, because we didn't want it to take over our life completely. When couples are talking with each other in the early days after a cancer diagnosis, how can they establish trust, define roles and soothe each other's fears and worries without letting it upend daily life?

Dr. Alise Bartley: Cancer—or any long-term health crisis—steals our power. When you receive a diagnosis, your sense of your own power shifts. You've lost control. When there is no imminent crisis and we are moving forward in life, we rarely think about how vulnerable we'd become if we were faced with a challenging illness. But if or when it happens, as the patient, you have to ask yourself what you can do to regain some of that power and agency. It can be really difficult, especially in the beginning, when you may not even know what you need.

As a caregiver to a partner, there can be awkward silences at the beginning of this process since we are still in disbelief—and we need to be! But the most important question you can ask your loved one is very simple: "What do you need?" And to be clear, it's not, "What can I do for you?" Because that's more about you. Asking what they need allows the space for them to share more freely, even if what they need goes beyond what you might be able to provide personally. The greatest gift you can give to your partner may just be to truly listen.

In general, couples should think about defining some parameters—I don't really like the word "boundaries" because it's so overused—for how and when they'll talk about and deal with their illness. There's no denying it will take an important place in their life together, but they don't want to build the next phase of their relationship on top of the crisis. Instead, the goal should be to lean on the strength of the partnership to support them both through it.

RJS: Should every couple navigating a serious illness get a therapist?

DAB: This depends on the couple. When there is a lot of trust and intimacy in the relationship, it's an easier ask if one person wants to speak to a therapist, because it isn't perceived as a threat to that intimacy.

Therapy offers a number of great benefits, including opening a safe, judgment-free space in which to explore all your feelings or to have a conversation that might be difficult to start. A good therapist can also help you create structures and define those parameters I mentioned, which are key to not letting a crisis consume you. And we know that structure is really important to managing the stress and anxiety that can come with the chaos of a diagnosis.

RJS: How can couples find the right therapist? Should they speak to their oncologist? What are some important things to consider?

DAB: You should certainly talk with your medical team. In the same way as when you're choosing an oncologist, you should sense an immediate and real rapport with any counselor or therapist you're considering. I always say that whenever you interact with your therapist, you should feel that you're their one and only patient, their primary concern. Even if they're busy. Even if they're a superstar in their field. We know that trust in your therapist plays the most important role in the success of your overall experience,[1] so it's really key to follow your instincts.[2]

More specifically, look for someone who has a background in chronic illness and consider bringing them on early in your process if you can, as the relationship can be most useful if your therapist continues with you throughout the journey.

RJS: What about the differences between women and men? Is there anything to consider? During Melissa's medical crisis, I had to do a lot of things I never expected, and if I were to credit one person with helping me do that, it would be my mother. She had an incredible inner strength that made her able to meet any challenge or problem.

DAB: In our society, women are socialized as caregivers. I once had a patient who'd had a heart attack. She had been hosting a Fourth of July party and ignored serious symptoms because she didn't want to inconvenience her guests. If you are a woman stepping into the patient role, you may feel guilty or that you're losing your purpose. Instead, think of it as gently setting down that role just for now. For the time being, you need to break away from being the constant caregiver and give yourself the attention and space to heal.

The same can be said for men who are suddenly thrust into the role of patient or caregiver. Changing roles create uncertainty and can bring anxiety, unease or feelings of being overwhelmed. Again, creating structure and being gentle with yourself during these transitions is key. Therapy can offer a lot of relief as well as proactive solutions for managing this new chapter and continuing to thrive as a couple.[3]

A Special Note to Men Becoming Caregivers to Partners Experiencing a Long-Term Medical Crisis:

While male and female caregivers both confront many of the same responsibilities and experience additional pressures, the fact that women in our society are more

continued on the next page

socialized as caregivers has an impact on their ability to handle those responsibilities over the long term in the context of a relationship. That is not necessarily the case for men.

One 2009 study of 550 couples "confirmed earlier research that put the overall divorce or separation rate among cancer patients at 11.6 percent, similar to the population as a whole. However, researchers were surprised by the difference in separation and divorce rates by gender. The rate when the woman was the patient was 20.8 percent compared to 2.9 percent when the man was the patient."

These striking statistics are worth mentioning here—not because they paint a negative portrait of men as caregivers, but because they indicate that men, when thrust into a medical crisis with their partner, may need additional support. If you know this early on, you can be prepared to find and take advantage of counseling services, spiritual guidance and other techniques to help manage these unique demands.

CHAPTER TAKEAWAYS:

- Choose your medical team based on your own situation and needs
- Think about your roles and tasks in the context of the illness
- Consider your budget and make any necessary plans or adjustments
- Communicate clearly with your healthcare professionals
- Prioritize deepening communicating and supporting each other as partners
- Expect the unexpected, and stay strong

**"WE HAVE TWO EARS
AND ONLY ONE MOUTH
SO WE CAN LISTEN
TWICE AS MUCH
AS WE SPEAK."**

—Epictetus

Chapter 3
TAKING GOOD CARE

Darling,

Do you remember all the times we sang together in the car on our way to your treatment appointments? I was always trying to come up with a playlist of songs that would light up your smile and get you tapping your toes.

You told me in the beginning that you wanted our sweet life to continue, even in the face of this serious threat. You didn't want to lose the essence of what we were. You wanted music and lunches together and watching fun movies on our couch. It was what I wanted, too—in fact, I wanted to make your life even sweeter than it had been before.

And although you were the one dealing with nausea, your lovely hair falling out and exhaustion from all the toxic chemicals deployed in your body to battle your disease, you always gently reminded me to take care of myself.

It's true that we cried sometimes, but we mostly laughed and reminisced. In your eyes from time to time, especially at night, I saw a flicker of fear. Those moments tore me up inside. I knew I didn't have the power to personally cure your cancer, but I was sure as hell going to make you laugh and forget your troubles for a few moments whenever I could.

It was a wonderful life, filled with sweetness. Thank you, my love.

Bob

PRACTICAL ADVICE

Dealing with cancer feels like a job you never wanted: endless calls and emails, test results with words and numbers you don't understand, frustrating letters from your insurance provider and other run-around processes. It can also just be monotonous, with lots of time spent traveling and waiting around in doctors' offices and exam rooms, yet there's no alternative. It's a job you can't quit, even if you're not sure when, if ever, it will get easier. So, you dig in and you just get it done, but even more than most jobs, cancer is completely exhausting, physically and mentally—not just for the patient, but for the caregiver as well. You need to pace yourself and prioritize rest.

Taking "good" care of your partner and yourself is not as straightforward as it might seem. Almost everyone I know whose partner is in treatment focuses all their caregiving energy exclusively on their partner because, well, they're the one who is sick. We see ourselves, the caregivers, as not needing or deserving much, and we absolutely do not want to complain. For the moment, we're healthy, so what do we have to complain about?

Melissa and I found a really good balance, but to do so, we had to talk about it and keep each other's needs in mind. Here's some of what I learned as a caregiver over the course of our eight years in treatment.

Ask What Your Partner Needs Right Now

Sometimes when our loved one is in long-term treatment, we think what they need is the same routine, or that they'll want to be "cheered up" with festive gifts, balloons or music, when what they really want is a cocoon where they can be cozy and quiet while their body repairs itself. Other times, they may have a lot more energy and want to be more active. Focus on their needs rather than what you can do for them—it will help them feel heard, and it may provide clues to other resources you can seek.

Add Happy Moments to Treatment Days

Melissa and I were always foodies, so whenever it made sense, I would pick a restaurant to stop at before or after her appointments. Sometimes it didn't make sense because she wasn't feeling well, but other times, it was the perfect way to remind ourselves we could still really enjoy life, despite the challenges we were facing. Other things we liked to do: watch home improvement shows on HGTV (plus plenty of tennis and golf!) or stop at a bookstore or the mall to do a bit of shopping.

Make Playlists

Cancer patients often have to sit for long periods, whether in a car or on a bus on the way to treatment, in treatment itself while drugs are administered or in the lobbies of medical offices while waiting to visit their doctors. Making thoughtful playlists of music, podcasts, audiobooks, streaming series or even YouTube videos for all that downtime is a lovely way to show you care and to brighten their day as they work toward healing. You may even want to invite friends and family to contribute to a playlist for a meaningful shared activity.

Delight Their Senses

Cancer patients are often cold, as they often lose weight or their hair as a result of their treatments. In those cases, a cozy blanket can be a wonderful gift, as can a pair of comfy pajamas or fluffy socks. If your loved one likes spa scents, put a candle or aroma diffuser in their room. Touch is another sense that is often overlooked: offer them a foot rub with peppermint oil, a massage or a manicure appointment. In our case, there were times when Melissa was too sick to go to a salon, but since I knew she always loved to have beautiful nails, I found a mobile manicurist who could come to our house. On those days, we would sit outside while she had her toes and nails done as a special treat, and it really lifted her spirits.

Senses are everything. Serve food that they like right now. It may not be exactly what you'd eat, and it may vary from what they used to like to eat, but try to honor their wishes. Their body may be craving new flavors as it deals with the hardship of disease.

Reinforce Their Self-Esteem

Nothing ruins your confidence like losing your hair in clumps or dropping so much weight that your great outfits hang on you like curtains. Cancer can also make workouts difficult, and that can cause a drop in endorphins that feels like depression for someone who exercises regularly. To help boost their spirits, take the time to notice and appreciate your partner's beauty and style.

Melissa was devastated by the loss of her hair, yet she chose to shave it off before it all fell out. We got her a gorgeous wig, and I made sure to tell her that I really liked it (I did!). When her fashionable friends (who knew nothing about her sickness) also complimented her hair, it filled her sails again and she glowed.

Work on Little Projects Together

Look through photos, or make a printed album of birthdays or friends' get-togethers. I have always loved those digital photo frames, and since we had so many photos on our phones and cameras, I decided to put digital frames all over the house to play happy memories. This was a big hit with Melissa, and honestly, I still look at them nearly every single day.

Your project could be anything. Plan for a bathroom renovation or a new color of paint in the living room. Make a mood board to inspire your next vacation together on the beach, at a dude ranch or in a faraway city like Paris or Tokyo. Look toward the future together, and make it sweet.

Don't Force Activities

Even if it's New Year's Eve, your wedding anniversary or even your partner's birthday, they may not be up for whatever you're planning. Gentle coaxing is okay, but no means no. The tiredness and the sadness that sometimes accompany cancer can squash the desire to see people, celebrate or even have sex with a beloved partner. In these cases, wait until they're stronger, and find other ways to make happy moments. They'll love you all the more for your understanding and tenderness.

Avoid Big Surprises

This goes along with the point just above. When dealing with cancer, even a person who is normally spontaneous and up for anything may need more notice and approval over having visitors or doing activities that might otherwise be delightful, unexpected adventures. To give them a break, offer ideas instead of concrete plans. Visitors can be especially tricky. Some people love to have friends and family around for comfort, support and a sense of normalcy, while others just need to "nest" and rest during treatment.

Be as Flexible as You Can

There is no better training for bending like a willow branch than having to deal with illness. Just when you think you can take a weekend away, go out to the theater, see friends or even just sit at the dinner table and eat a real meal, things come up. It can be incredibly frustrating and even annoying at times, but the sooner you learn to let things slide and to be willing to pivot, the better it will be for the both of you.

Help Them Work Out in a Way That Works

"In a way that works" is the key phrase here. Melissa liked the recumbent bike, the one where you sort of sit back and really just use your legs. Even a few minutes made a big difference in her mood and her strength levels. But you have to let your partner lead. Trying to force them into exercising is not helpful, but you can ask what they might like and help make it possible, even if it means setting up a mini-gym in your living room or bedroom.

If You're Your Partner's Caregiver, Don't Forget to Take Care of Yourself

And by the way, that's an order. It's such a cliché and caregivers struggle to heed this advice, but I promise you, it can make all the difference. If you look at the most successful CEOs in the world, they often credit daily exercise, a healthy diet or meditation with giving them the strength and mental clarity to deal with extreme pressure, super-tight deadlines and crisis situations.

This is true of cancer caregivers, too. You don't have to be an Olympic athlete or run a marathon, but you should try to get some walking or stretching in every day and prioritize your nutrition, sleep and even quiet time whenever you can.

Note: This is not selfish. It's *self-preparation* for being a great caregiver who has the energy and bandwidth to do what it takes for the person they love.

HELP FROM THE EXPERTS

Not everyone is aware of integrative medicine, but in a nutshell, it's about treating the *whole* person—not just with medication, but by looking at other aspects of their life and health as well to give them the best foundation for healing.

Melissa and I found the integrative approach to be fulfilling and productive. Our treatment plan was carefully crafted and tailored by our team, all of whom were setting us up for success. In fact, as a result of our experience, I created an endowment for the integrative medicine department at University Hospital of Cleveland, and I continue to work with them to expand awareness and access, so I wanted to prioritize the subject in this chapter.

To explain the benefits and possibilities of integrative healthcare, I chose a brilliant physician, Santosh Rao, whom I met in the process of putting together this book. He is a dedicated and passionate doctor who is open to ideas, believes in seeing and treating the whole person during their illness and is eager to help others take advantage of integrative care.

INTEGRATIVE ONCOLOGY AND CREATING A PERSONALIZED TREATMENT PLAN:
A Conversation with Santosh Rao, MD, Medical Director of a Nationally Recognized Integrative Oncology Program and Medical Oncologist, President of the Soceity for Integrative Oncology

Robert J. Shearer: I'm so happy to be having this conversation with you, because I want to help people understand the importance of integrative medicine—and more specifically, integrative oncology and how it can improve their outcomes of serious illnesses. Could you start by just explaining what its components are and what its benefits can be?

Dr. Santosh Rao: Yes. It can seem hard to describe exactly what integrative oncology is, so let me first start with a definition that was put together by an organization I'm a part of, the Society for Integrative Oncology:

"Integrative oncology is a patient-centered, evidence-informed field of cancer care that utilizes mind and body practices, natural products and/or lifestyle modifications from different traditions alongside conventional cancer treatments. Integrative oncology aims to optimize health, quality of life and clinical outcomes across the cancer care continuum and to empower people to become active participants before, during and beyond cancer treatment."

The first thing to know is that in an integrative approach, we are supporting and empowering people and what they can do for themselves. In medicine, we often focus on treatment and not as much on what people can actually do on their own behalf. In learning more about how impactful this integrative approach is—not only for prevention but also post-diagnosis, in treatment and in survivorship—we know it matters what you do, your mindset, your lifestyle and whether you're optimistic or not. These things matter a lot. We aim to engage with all our patients on this holistic approach, because if we don't, we are missing an opportunity to help them.

Another thing to note is that there's a cultural aspect to people's needs and preferences when they're diagnosed. This is true all around the world. Cancer care looks different depending on how a person grew up, what they eat, even what they believe. To empower them, we need to approach their treatment specifically, and we need to take into account the whole person. What has helped them in the past? What practices are natural for them? There is wisdom in many cultures that can be difficult to fold into our traditional medicine.

And then it's important to mention that integrative therapy is becoming very popular, but it is not always well coordinated. It's key to combine complementary and conventional care for the best outcomes, but not every medical center or practice has the same offerings.

Also, there's a time and place for where you do what, and that all comes down to the patient and their disease. Let's say a patient is experiencing pain or anxiety, and treatment through acupuncture is working. Why would you give them a narcotic?

But on the flipside, there are times when folks want an alternative that isn't available. One example might be that a patient doesn't want to do certain hormonal treatments. They'd prefer to treat their disease naturally, but that option doesn't happen to exist in this case. There isn't scientific evidence for a replacement. We need to give good advice while taking into account the specifics of the situation, the stage of the disease and the science.

As to why I chose this path, it started a long time ago. I was interested in holistic medicine even before I chose to be a doctor. I was a biophysics major, but I developed an interest in yoga, meditation, Chinese medicine and Ayurveda. Without yet fully understanding medicine, I did an independent study, and it became a strong passion of mine. I felt there was something missing in terms of what we consider "health."

As I entered medicine and learned so many things, it was fascinating that we didn't spend a lot of time on health. We focused mainly on disease. Things are changing, and many in our field are interested in integrative oncology because it's impactful. We know that guiding people in exercise, nutrition, mindfulness and so on is important.

That was my spark: an affinity for traditional knowledge from varying cultures, self-healing, prevention and empowerment. That approach has carried through up until now.

RJS: For those who are wondering, is there a difference between integrative and alternative medicine?

DSR: Yes, there is actually a big difference. In fact, we navigate away from the term "alternative." "Integrative" means complementary and coordinated. It doesn't eschew conventional treatment, but rather is meant as a complement. "Alternative" means different, which is not at all the same thing.

Studies show if you abandon conventional medicine, you generally have worse outcomes. When patients ask me about "alternative" treatments, I say no. Our approach is: "What is evidence-based and scientifically proven?" Things that work would by their nature, not simply being alternative.

That said, there are many things that are now conventional that used to be alternative. Take, for example, how we treat ulcers. If 50 years ago someone had given a patient antibiotics for an ulcer, that would've been considered crazy. Now it's completely conventional.

The caveat to all this is that there is still more money in conventional medicine. The pharmaceutical industry has billions of dollars for research and development, and that's just not true for research into integrative medicine. They're not equal. The goal is to make integrative medicine practical and based on science—to use it to enhance care, not to try to create a sense of this or that opposing approach.

RJS: So, if you're in cancer treatment, how do you make sure you have that integrative or holistic approach in your overall treatment plan? Is it something you can ask for? Should you screen your medical center or your physician to find out what options are available?

DSR: Integrative oncology is an evolving field, and it's not available everywhere, although it's rapidly growing. Studies looking at large cancer centers show that there is an increasing presence of integrative oncology.

But even where integrative care is available, the offerings differ in different places. If you're considering an integrative approach, it's a very personal question. How important is it to you and where do you live? As an example, San Francisco, New York and other major metropolitan areas will likely have a number of options, but if you live in a more rural setting, there may not be much choice in terms of finding a medical center with an organized, integrative program.

Also, beyond where you live, depending upon the type of cancer and the stage or situation, screening your medical team for integrative options may not actually be your number one priority. But absolutely, you should ask what is available, and educate yourself so that you can make the right decision for you.

Even if you're not able to access integrative treatment through your medical team, they will likely be able to point you toward resources. And then through the internet, there are options for online education, communities and even advocates.

And of course, some modalities, including acupuncture, yoga and massage, for example, are available nearly everywhere, so you can put together your own complementary therapies. But do make sure to let your physician know about anything you're planning.

RJS: Who leads the team when integrative medicine is part of the treatment? Is it the main oncologist or is there a separate doctor or team who collaborates? Is an integrative approach available everywhere or is it important to ask about it?

DSR: Since it's different depending on where you receive care, let's look at one example. For a cancer patient, it's very important to have a coordinated plan. That means that, for example, the surgeon, the radiation doctor and the integrative physician are taking a team approach. In this case, it's important for someone to be the "lead", depending on the cancer and the stage.

Most important, though, is that the doctors are in conversation and are working together collaboratively, not sending mixed messages. In our case, we'll exchange feedback, then make a plan that might add music therapy, stress management and exercise in addition to conventional treatment. We work together whether I am leading the team, as sometimes happens, or I'm consulting with the lead physician and other doctors.

RJS: When Melissa was treated at UH, we also did some of these things. I called it a holistic approach. Acupuncture didn't work, because she hated needles, so we did yoga, music therapy and massage, plus we had worked with a nutritionist even before Melissa's illness. But I'm wondering, is talking with a psychologist part of an integrative treatment plan?

DSR: It depends. Rather than saying which specific modalities are "in" or "out" of an integrative plan, I'd emphasize that integrative medicine is a philosophy and an approach to care rather than a "we own this part of the care" stance.

Depending upon where you are and what your program offers, the psychologist you see might be a part of the integrative team, or they might be a third party who is providing that care but who coordinates with the other members of your team.

In an integrative approach to treatment, our goal is to empower our patients and help them understand their resources. At UH, everyone on the team is aiming to reduce toxicity and complications and to improve results.

RJS: What else would you like to share about integrative medicine to help people understand it as an essential part of their treatment plan?

DSR: This is an area of medicine that meets people where they are, that takes into account everything from their lifestyle and spirituality to their preferences. In the past, it has been under-emphasized.

I've been doing this for 10 years, and while there are courses and books on the topic, it's still a journey as a physician. How do we engage patients on their own personal beliefs, their lifestyle? If you talk to them, you'll find they want to share, and they have lots of questions. They want partners to help them navigate.

It's all about personalizing things, self-affirming care, empowering patients, promoting self-healing and self-awareness. We're focused on the science, and these approaches are now in our major guidelines. There are opportunities to help with a wide range of issues, including fatigue, depression and pain.

The approach has changed from the view from, "If it's available, okay," to now being considered, in my opinion, standard-of-care. The research is building. When you have options that are non-toxic and/or less expensive, they are now considered a first or second choice for some symptoms.

The conversation is changing now to, "How do we make this available to those who need it?" This is a big part of what I'm working on. If we find these treatments helpful, money shouldn't be the barrier.

I've talked to people all over the United States and around the world about these issues. The Navajo people, for example, sometimes have to drive 300 miles to get to a cancer center. So many people don't have access to good nutrition, or they can't afford massage or acupuncture. How do we meet those needs? How do we deliver guideline-driven care?

The next step is how we access the resources to make that available and to continue to do research. What's the best option? And then if it works, how do we make it standard-of-care and universal?

Medical centers are working hard to meet this need—firstly, because patients want it, and secondly, because it's matched with research.

The question is: How do you weave in these complementary therapies? A part of my role is to educate my colleagues so that they can amplify the message. For example, I want the nurses in our center to be empowered to educate our patients. The goal is to infuse holistic care and wellness, to blend it with the traditional model and bring it into the standard of care.

RJS: I'm a firm believer. Thank you for sharing all this info. Not a lot is said about it. Could you just talk a bit about "lifestyle oncology" for those who don't know the term?

DSR: There are many things that fall under the umbrella of integrative medicine. There's functional medicine, lifestyle medicine and the like. They all blend in different ways. At UH, we partner with the American College of Lifestyle Medicine. Lifestyle, meaning what you do on a regular basis, obviously can have a strong influence on health in general and on outcomes, but if a patient has advanced cancer or is going through chemotherapy, for example, we might choose to focus on dietary needs such as calorie and protein requirements, maintaining physical activity and stress management rather than other adjustments.

As for prevention, we want to educate patients about lifestyle and stress management, whether it's before a cancer diagnosis or after treatment in survivorship. In fact, we're starting a program with a group of providers over multiple weeks to educate our patients.

It's not that we're the only ones who can talk about lifestyle. We don't need to own that conversation, but in a large program like ours, the more people who talk about it, the better.

Part of our approach will be to engage with our underserved population and to work with our community partners. The challenge is the bad outcomes that occur when people can't afford their care or prevention. Poor diet, stress and trauma, even in childhood, can all have an effect.

Prevention is complex and takes a lot of work and team effort. This is my personal passion. As the old maxim says, "An ounce of prevention is worth a pound of cure." We want people to have their health, enjoy life and reduce suffering. Anything we can do up front and implement in advance is the intelligent thing to do.

CHAPTER TAKEAWAYS:

- Ask your partner what they need right now and really listen
- Infuse your life together with extra sweetness and small gestures to create joy even during a difficult time
- Be flexible with plans and activities
- Ask your medical team about integrative medicine and your treatment plan
- Prioritize your own nutrition, exercise and sleep to support your caregiving

"THE FIRST TWO RULES OF BECOMING A CAREGIVER:

1. **IT WILL BE DIFFICULT.**
2. **IT WILL BE WORTH IT."**

—Laura Finney

Chapter 4

OFF THE BEATEN PATH

Melissa,

Do you remember our visits to the psychologist? They weren't always easy.

The main thing that seemed to concern the various doctors we met was the fact that you didn't want to share the news of your cancer with anyone outside of a very tight and trusted circle. You did not want to "work through the issue" in therapy. You were totally clear on what you wanted.

Once, the doctor even called to say she was worried for me and what the stress of keeping quiet about your illness might do to me. I remember just thinking, "My beautiful wife has her own strong opinions. This is her decision, and I will support whatever she wants." It didn't mean that I always agreed with you, but I knew and respected that you were the decider. So, we put psychotherapy to the side and focused on other options.

We were completely aligned about using a wide variety of additional therapies to keep you strong and help you through. We were already big believers in the importance of chiropractic and nutrition, so we just upped our commitment there. Since we both loved massage, that became another resource and comfort as well.

The important thing is we always considered complementary medicine a valuable part of your treatment, and we sought out experts to put a plan together that would give your body a solid foundation to be as strong as possible, to keep you feeling well along the way.

Since the additional therapies had a positive effect on your overall health, and I know you agree, I want to tell others what our process was like.

My goal is to encourage them to seek out things to keep them feeling well and comfortable, too, just as we did for you.

Love,

Bob

PRACTICAL ADVICE

Everyone has opinions about their own care or their approach to caregiving. Some people are more comfortable with traditional medicine, while others believe in leveraging other practices to serve the larger objective of healing.

More and more, practices like chiropractic and acupuncture are becoming accepted as valuable and effective options, and Melissa and I spent a lot of time with our healthcare team creating the right mix for us.

For example, I do still occasionally laugh about "the acupuncture adventure" we had one day. Although I took Melissa to the practitioner's office, they never managed to get a single needle in her. Everyone who knew her knew that needles, wherever optional, were out of the question. It was simply wishful thinking on my part, but in seeing how uncomfortable it made her, I let it go, and we focused elsewhere.

I hope the suggestions below will support your well-being throughout your own process, whether you're the patient or the caregiver.

Do Your Research

First, ask your medical team about a "whole person" approach to your medical challenges. See what they offer and what they recommend. Ask friends who may have been through a similar experience if they have providers they really like. Educate yourself on what the options are and read reviews of any practitioners or products you may be considering.

Give Special Focus to Diet and Movement

Many experts agree that food and even supplements can be tools to healing and can support your body in so many ways. You may choose to alter your diet—to focus more on plant-based foods, for example—or to eliminate certain foods that are inflammatory or processed. It's the same for gentle movement or your favorite physical activity. With a regular practice of working out or moving, you may find your mood lifting and your body feeling more resilient.

Treat Your Body Well

If you have the means to integrate them into your plan, this may mean getting an aromatherapy massage, doing other complementary treatments if they appeal to you or even considering reiki.

Consider the Benefits of Traditional Eastern Treatments

Acupuncture, for example, wasn't for Melissa—but I absolutely love it, and it has helped me with a variety of issues. Be open to possibilities, and if your team (or a trusted friend) recommends something new to you, maybe give it a try and see how it makes you feel.

Lean on Your Culture

Think about the tools you have to help you support your healing. Whether that's your faith, a family tradition for using herbs and plants to support your health or prioritizing a yoga practice, build layers of well-being into your everyday life.

Keep Your Medical Team in the Loop

Even herbal supplements or dietary choices may impact certain medications or treatments, so you must make sure your doctor is aware of anything you're considering that falls outside your more traditional treatment plan. Make your healthcare team your partners in helping you craft an approach that takes your medical needs and well-being into account.

HELP FROM THE EXPERTS

What exactly does a "holistic" or "complementary" treatment plan look like? It's different for each person and family, and you should feel empowered to discuss your preferences, priorities and questions with the leaders of your medical team to create a combination of elements that's right for you.

In this chapter, we'll focus on talks with two experts on different aspects of complementary care. First, since I'm such a strong believer in chiropractic and nutrition, I've enlisted the help of Kelly Farrell-Emley, an expert in both fields who is a good friend and was to Melissa as well.

After that, I'll share a discussion with Bob Kaleal, a personal trainer and sports therapist I learned about through my dear friend Neil, whose wife said she benefited greatly from Bob's physical treatments while she battled cancer.

Even if you're not sure about complementary treatments, keep your mind and heart open and see if any of it resonates with you as you put together your own plan.

NUTRITION AND COMPLEMENTARY MEDICINE IN A HOLISTIC APPROACH TO TREATING SERIOUS ILLNESS: Guidance from Doctor of Chiropractic and Nutritional Wellness Expert Kelly Farrell-Emley

Robert J. Shearer Could you help us understand how natural health practices can work in collaboration with an individual medical program for better outcomes?

Dr. Kelly Farrell-Emley: When it comes to our health, it's extremely important that we have a strong and balanced foundation. Most chronic disease starts with an imbalance, so being able to identify and correct or improve system disruptions is crucial. We want to reduce chronic stress, both for disease prevention and for optimal health.

A great starting point is a thorough panel. There are other tests as well, but since cancer patients are generally getting regular reports, we find it very helpful to review them as a tool for finding imbalances. Overall, everyone will respond better to treatment if their bodily systems are functioning well.

RJS: I know that in addition to being a doctor of chiropractic, you have a broad expertise in using nutrition to support patients in cancer treatment. You helped Melissa so much over the years, and she really credited nutrition as improving her overall well-being. What is the most important thing to know about nutrition when you are battling a long-term disease such as cancer?

DKF-E: When it comes to cancer, people are doing a variety of interventions, such as radiation and chemotherapy, which can wreak havoc on the body, weaken immunity and the like. Choosing the best quality foods available—meaning organic, GMO-free and chemical-free foods—is a way to boost your system's resources.

We also believe that supplementing nutritious foods with essential vitamins can help keep the body stronger and restore balance in the system, so using whole-food, nutritional supplements is one of our recommended foundations.

RJS: We used their supplements even prior to Melissa being sick. They have no GMOs and no synthetic ingredients, which was important to us.

DKF-E: Yes, the whole-food supplement concept is becoming much more popular, especially because it's completely natural. A lot of vitamins in the supermarket are synthetic, with the chemical properties of a given vitamin. But they're often not the complete vitamin. It's the completeness of the vitamin and the way it interacts with your body that we are looking for.

The idea is to use natural means to support the body's functions as it works on healing. In cancer patients specifically, there may be multiple systems in dysfunction at the same time. Examples may include liver or thyroid problems, for example. Our philosophy is that we're giving the body the basics it needs to help it fight.

The key thing to note is that in our practice, we are not treating or curing cancer. We're focused on making the body stronger. The stronger the system is, the better it can engage, attack and heal.

RJS: What if your doctor or medical team doesn't believe in a more integrative approach to your health? Should you share what you're doing with them anyway? As in, should you tell them you're considering taking nutritional supplements, for example, or that you want to try acupuncture or other additional treatments?

DKF-E: I think in this day and age, doctors are becoming more aware of complementary medicine—acupuncture, chiropractic and other practices. But yes, it's very important to have that dialogue with your doctor. If they are resistant to integrative treatments, why? Could their hesitancy be based on personal beliefs? Talk with them, and don't be afraid to ask what is influencing their opinions.

RJS: When it comes to eating "healthy" while you're in treatment for a serious illness, what if your appetite is not great or certain foods just seem unappealing? What if you're craving less healthy foods or even junk food or sugar for example?

DKF-E: Honestly, cravings are a very normal thing that happens. As much as possible, you just want to make sure that you're favoring quality, organic foods and reducing the chemical burden in all the foods you choose.

As an example, you can either buy organic, minimally processed chicken, or factory chicken that, as a result of its processing, has been effectively saturated in chemicals. Knowing the quality of your foods, their source and how they came into the package is crucial.

If you find you have little or no appetite, you'll have to be very strategic with your foods. You need to increase the quality and density of calories and nutrition in the foods you're eating—nut butters, seed bread and other organic whole foods. Then for supplements, if you opt for the whole-food supplement method we discussed above, you can find tablets, capsules and sometimes even chewable wafers or powders, depending upon your nutritional goals. In most cases, whole-food supplements won't make you feel nauseous or sick.

RJS: Sugar was always a concern for us, because Melissa really loved chocolate. We tried hard to stay away from anything sweet and from sugary additives in sauces and breads, for example. It's true though that, from time to time, after she'd had a chemo treatment and her appetite was weak, I'd get her a milkshake, because I knew it was one thing she'd really like.

DKF-E: Yes, sometimes you need those extra calories as well. But it has to be said: sugar is bad for all types of disease. We strongly recommend eliminating it or reducing it as much as possible from your diet, especially if you are in treatment. Now, though, there are all kinds of sweeteners or forms of sugar you can substitute like monkfruit and Stevia, for example. Companies are even making cake mixes that are totally organic, with healthy flour and no sugar.

The thing is, sugar weakens the immune system and can feed infection. With a high-sugar diet, many experts believe cancer cells can grow even faster. The bad news is, when you eat too much sugar, you increase candida in your gut, and that creates powerful cravings in your body that your brain has a very hard time overruling. The good news is if you progressively eat less sugar, you'll start to crave it less. Additionally, supplements can help to rid the gut of candida and help the body overcome sugar cravings.

RJS: Sometimes adding in supplements, shopping for totally organic products and cooking from scratch can seem like a tall order, financially and even timewise, when you're juggling medical appointments, work and family. Do you have any tips for managing costs and/or making the process of preparing foods easier?

DKF-E: Once you get into knowing your brands and labels, controlling costs and even organizing, your shopping will be easier. It will take a little research, but you can find healthy organic foods at a cheaper price. Then, to help with time management, you can set up a delivery service every week and just keep a reorder list. And I always suggest making a recipe book or box that you can quickly glance at for inspiration and meal prep.

RJS: What about chiropractic and cancer? Is it safe? What kind of symptoms or troubles can it help with during treatment? Is there anything special we should consider before adding this into our overall health program?

DKF-E: Chiropractic is immune-upregulating in and of itself. Studies prove that when you get adjusted, there is a boost to your immune system. Also, neurologically, it reactivates the system and gets it talking to itself for better performance.

There may be inflammation and/or toxicity from the cancer treatment or due to past lifestyle issues. Chiropractic adjustment increases blood flow and can remove toxins. Done twice per month, for example, it can also be very effective for pain. It makes you feel better in your body.

Before chiropractic treatment, it's important to determine that there is no bone weakness. We evaluate everyone very carefully, discuss their pain and their overall health. There are many types of adjustment possible, so we tailor our treatment to the individual and where they are right now.

An individual treatment plan is the key to success with nutritional programs, chiropractic and other integrative approaches. Find a well-respected team who will listen to your concerns, look at you as an individual and help you combine methods to boost your body's strength so that you're in a better position to heal.

EXERCISE, MOVEMENT AND CANCER: Ideas, Tips and What You Need to Know from Bob Kaleal, Sports Therapist and Personal Trainer

Robert J. Shearer: Could you share a bit of your background and how you came to work with patients navigating cancer and other serious illnesses?

Bob Kaleal: After a kind of rocky childhood, I was a bit of a lost young man. I decided to go to paramedic school, and there I started to understand the body. I found my passion for helping others and continued on that path, eventually studying massage therapy, sports massage and advanced neuromuscular therapy. I remember at one point, I was working with my grandfather, training thoroughbred horses in the very early morning and then going to school later in the day. I knew this was what I wanted to do.

Later, I applied for sports medicine school at Baldwin Wallace College. I graduated, then got two master's degrees at Cleveland State. That's when it all started to come together. I wanted to take an approach of combining holistic health and wellness with movement and love and energy and what science has proven—you have to move, get endorphins, all the good stuff.

When I opened my first little gym, I signed up for a cancer wellness/fitness program. In Cleveland in 1999, people weren't as open-minded to functional medicine, and I wanted to shake things up, but it was difficult. I didn't give up, just kept going.

Then in 2006–2007, I started working with a group of post-chemo cancer kids, ages six to 16, at Rainbow Babies and Children's Hospital. It was my world opening up. We had eight kids in that first group, and I said to myself, "There's something here." I'm still working with kids today, among a variety of other ages of patients navigating different medical crises.

RJS: As an exercise expert and personal trainer, you've done a lot of work with people who are in the middle of a serious illness, including people who are being treated for cancer. I also know you've done research around this topic. What have you learned about how exercise interacts with and affects chemotherapy, for example?

BK: When people are sick, especially with a serious illness like cancer, let's face it: It's hard for them to take care of themselves. They don't have energy, they don't feel good in their bodies. There is so much in the aggressive treatments and chemicals that, while important, also creates problems.

It's my mission to help to push the drugs through the body, using movement and vibration therapy, for example. I've also introduced clients to dancing, even boxing. I'm always looking for the thing that will click with them.

RJS: What is vibration therapy? As you know, Melissa never had the good fortune to work with you, but you've helped some of our very close friends, and I think a lot of people may never have heard about this method.

BK: Vibration therapy circulates blood flow all through the body. For ease in imagining it, it's like when you jump on a mini trampoline. That motion is called rebounding, which in effect is vibration.

In the case of patients I work with, I have them lie down, often while they're in treatment or just after a treatment. I might start on one leg or foot, rocking them or shaking them—at a very low intensity, but somewhat rapidly. Then, I stretch them and work on another area of the body. The thought is to push the chemo through and then let your body eliminate it.

RJS: Are people generally open to this, considering that it's not super well known?

BK: What I've found out is that some spouses or significant others don't believe in this approach, and certainly some doctors are not on board. They say, "Oh, that can't work." But I've had support from some nurses, and I've personally seen some of my clients really have a better experience. Of course, this is just my own practice.

One client was in her 30s and had brain cancer. With the combination of her treatment and our working together, she went into remission, then actually got pregnant and had a baby boy before she died at age 37.

RJS: I'm a big believer in a holistic approach. I've been using massage therapy for 35 years. I'm in Arizona now, and I've started Thai massage. It's really wonderful.

BK: Yes, Thai massage is great.

RJS: With Melissa, I was limited as to who could work with us, because she didn't want anyone to know she was sick. But we had a good friend who had experience with massaging cancer patients, so we confided in her. She helped us a great deal, and I definitely saw an improvement in Melissa's mood, appetite and general wellness.

But specifically for cancer patients who are undergoing chemotherapy, what types of exercises do you recommend? Is cardio more important than weight training, for example?

BK: With cancer, heavy bouts of chemo deplete energy, so we can't do typical strength training where you are basically tearing down muscles and rebuilding stronger. With cancer, you do a modified form. It could be just rubber band training, for example. We get the heart rate up, because heavy breathing promotes faster blood flow, and we want that.

In between short sets of cardio movement, even just marching in place helps—you can do chest presses or bicep curls with bands, for example. Then, you want to do balance work. At the end of a workout, I love to repeat cardio for the whole body for 30-45 minutes. Every day, four to five days per week, medium-to-low intensity until remission, and then we turn it up a level.

RJS: How do you feel about yoga and pilates during cancer treatment?

BK: I love it. Modified yoga is great, because some people may be frail or weak. I like to build confidence with low-intensity programs tailored to each patient. That includes the mindset and nutrition, too. It's all connected.

RJS: What if someone is very active—let's say you have a runner or someone who plays tennis a lot. Should they continue to follow their routine as long as they feel well enough? Or should they plan for adjustments in their workouts and even their expectations as a part of organizing their treatments?

BK: There are people who know they're sick, yet they still fight the battle to maintain a high level of fitness, which can be good or bad. Then there are those who deny that they're really sick. They let their pride get the best of them, and in this case, not meeting expectations can really mess with their mental state.

I try to lower expectations just a little while still creating a fulfilling and challenging program. I just want to avoid injuries, even small strains or sprains with folks in chemo. The main thing is to stay nutrient-dense at all times and to respect your fatigue.

Sometimes we'll play half a game of tennis and then stop, go in the other room, stretch and do band work. We achieve the same output and still have the enjoyment of the sport, but without the increased potential for injury. If you're healthy and feeling good, then I won't stop you from doing what you love, but I may suggest we modify it in small but significant ways.

RJS: What advice would you have for those who want to create a home exercise space and a routine for themselves?

BK: I'm actually working on some really cool technological solutions to help folks create tailored programs via avatar technology and an application we're developing, and I even hold a number of patents. So I hope to have more to share on that soon.

But in the meantime, you can buy yourself home rubber bands, a mat and a mini-trampoline. If you can, try to find a personal trainer to help you. If not, look for an app with guided workouts and tailor them to your energy and strength levels. Medicine is crucial, but you need to focus on yourself as a whole person. That means movement and quality nutrition every single day.

We need to realize that these life-saving drugs can be even better if you put a program in place to help support them. Since we know that chemo causes some harm along with the good, our goal is to provide support with this solution.

RJS: What about a person who, before their diagnosis, was not really sporty or athletic? Would you still recommend they start to incorporate movement or exercise into their routine?

BK: Yes, yes and yes! Movement is key to good health. As they say, "A body in motion, stays in motion."

RJS: Often cancer treatment can make the patient really tired. Do you have any tips or exercise ideas for boosting energy, even if they're just lying in bed?

BK: Rebounding and vibration therapy are amazing. They provide energy and heighten the body's awareness. You need green drinks, berries and foods that are super-packed full of nutrition. The fatigue is a result of the chemo. Your body is being depleted, and your hair is falling out, so whatever you can do to boost your system and give your body strength and energy can help.

Talk to your doctor about solutions to help you have a bit more appetite and energy. Some patients will get a prescription for medications that can help, and I believe marijuana can be amazing for your body during cancer treatment. There are even those who support micro-dosing mushrooms. I'm not advocating any specific medications or drugs, I'm simply saying there are medicinal options and even gummies or droplets that can bring a level of energy. They are sometimes life-changing. Talk to your doctor to figure out what might work for you.

RJS: And for the caregiver of someone who is in cancer treatment, there can be so much stress and overwhelm that's often paired with exhaustion, especially if they are working during the day and helping to manage the care of their loved one. What would you suggest for them in terms of movement or exercise to help them stay healthy?

BK: You know what? I believe they should follow the same program. Eat, drink, stretch, move, support, laugh. Do it in tandem. It is sometimes so emotionally difficult, so if you can do it together, it may be good for you as a couple. As anyone who has a loved one going through a medical crisis knows, it can be really draining. I'm sure you might have been drained or feeling down, Bob—I can only imagine. What did you do for yourself?

RJS: Actually, I never felt down, but every morning I'd take our dogs out. I got outside and moved. In fact, this is why we started this book: to share our journey as a couple, and to try to help connect people to resources like you so they can know more earlier and really take advantage. Thank you so much for this conversation, and for the work you do.

BK: It's an honor. Thank you, Bob.

CHAPTER TAKEAWAYS:

- Consider combining natural health practices such as chiropractic, nutritional guidance and acupuncture with your medical treatment
- Focus on a healthy diet and some daily movement
- If you like, make movement a shared activity with your partner
- Focus on what works for you and don't worry about the rest
- Make sure to speak with your medical team about any complementary treatments you consider

"THE DOCTOR OF THE FUTURE WILL GIVE NO MEDICATION, BUT WILL INTEREST HIS PATIENTS IN THE CARE OF THE HUMAN FRAME, DIET, AND IN THE CAUSE AND PREVENTION OF DISEASE."

—Thomas Edison

Chapter 5
COPING WITH ILLNESS AS A COUPLE

Lovely Melissa,

In our life before your illness, we always decided things together.

Likewise, when we found out you had cancer, one of the first things we decided was that we would manage your illness as a team, using our entrepreneurial skills to look for answers and solutions. I do think our business experience really benefited us, because we had already weathered many stressful storms while building our company. We already had some of the skills we needed to handle difficult situations with calmness and presence of mind.

We were lucky, too, to have our dogs and our horses, who kept us connected with nature and joy. They really helped us cope, even if we might not have used that word back then.

You used your connection with art, beauty and culture to keep you centered and inspired, even during the most difficult moments. I loved watching movies with you and going for walks on the golf course. We always found a way to honor our belief that gratitude is everything.

You weren't just my lover and my wife. You were truly my best friend, and I was yours, through thick and thin and everything in between.

Bob

PRACTICAL ADVICE

Coping is a word that can seem kind of technical or even negative. When I used to think of it, I always saw it as having to just "deal" with a difficult situation. But on my journey with Melissa, I discovered that coping is really all about self-knowledge and reflection and creating strategies that help us through life, in good times and in challenging times.

The concept can mean dealing with something uncomfortable or difficult in real time or even after the fact, but developing coping skills can also be a preventative practice of amassing ideas and alternatives to have ready for whenever you need them.

Have you ever taken time to think about coping strategies that might work for you? I hope you and your partner will find this chapter helpful as you continue to support each other.

Tell Them You Love Them

In a crisis, there is nothing like the reassurance of love and support to lift spirits and build resilience. It's so important. I highly recommend sharing these things with your partner every single day that you're here, and telling them that you love them very much.

Do Things Together Outside of Treatment Times and Appointments

I've mentioned this before, but during a long illness, when things can be stressful and tiring, it is easy to let couple time and date nights slip and to prioritize the medical side of things more than the emotional connection you share. Melissa and I made a point of doing even more together—watching movies, playing with the dogs, eating out when we could—and you know what? It was wonderful, and it strengthened our bond beyond anything we could've imagined.

Respect Your Partner's Boundaries

This will be different for every couple, but be sure to listen when your partner tells you something is important to them, or when they share things that upset them or just plain don't like. Melissa didn't want to tell anyone about her illness, and I accepted that. She didn't like needles, so I didn't force things on the acupuncture, even though I believed in it and thought it would help her.

This can be difficult if you don't agree with your partner's wishes or priorities. I'd encourage you to go ahead and make your case, but then listen and treat their response with the utmost care and respect.

Stay In the Now as Much as You Can

The easiest way to get really stressed out during a battle with a serious medical issue is to think about the past or the future. You can beat yourself up about what you should've done or what you didn't do, or you can spend your time inventing scary stories about the future. I don't recommend either.

Keep yourself grounded in the moment and consider starting a meditation practice, or just sit quietly and breathe deeply for a few minutes each day. This can help keep your mood balanced and make you feel g stronger, to deal with whatever may come. It may also have a calming effect on your partner.

Agree to Avoid Any Unnecessary Quarrels

I recently heard a great piece of marriage advice from a wildly successful self-made entrepreneur married to another wildly successful self-made entrepreneur. They agreed early in their marriage to evaluate every possible issue as it came up on a scale of one to 10. If any irritation or misunderstanding rated less than a seven on that scale, they would just let it go and forget about it. If it was a seven or above, they committed to dealing with it openly and respectfully. What a great idea—if it's less than a seven, just let it go!

HELP FROM THE EXPERTS

What's so interesting to me in having the opportunity to talk with an expert like Dr. Alise Bartley is that when we're in crisis as a couple, there is such an advantage to actively shoring up the foundation of our relationship to make sure it's as strong as possible.

But everything she shares in this conversation and throughout the book is just plain good advice for being in a relationship at any time at all, and for taking the time to prioritize the health of not just your body but a deep connection with your partner. Coping during an illness is a skill we must cultivate.

At the end of the discussion, you'll find a great worksheet of ideas for creating coping skills that are positive, productive and work for you.

BUILDING YOUR TOOLKIT OF COPING SKILLS: More Advice from Dr. Alise Bartley

Robert J. Shearer: What exactly is "coping," and how can skills and techniques help you when you need them?

Dr. Alise Bartley: I define coping as not changing the situation, but figuring out how to adapt to what is happening to you or around you. So many times in life, things happen that we can't change, but how do we want to respond to those situations? Our response is the most important and powerful part of how we can transcend a situation.

When we're coping, we're trying to figure out how to free ourselves from what is happening, from what it means. When we're knee deep in our emotions, we can't always see that there is another way to respond. Having healthy coping skills empowers us to choose a response that will help us.

Of course, there are unhealthy coping strategies, too—like overeating, drinking too much and so on. But if you have access to a healthier approach, it gives you confidence that you can make it through."

RJS: I'd love to address specific situations where coping skills might really help. What if you're frustrated with something—your medical treatment, your partner not communicating, financial worries as a result of your needed medicines or your surgeries?

DAB: First and foremost, we have to honor our emotions. We tend to not allow ourselves to actually experience what we're experiencing, but we need to acknowledge what we're going through. We have to say, "Wow, I'm feeling really sad today," not just, "I'm fine, I'm fine."

Once we acknowledge those feelings, we should just be with them for a bit. We should sit in them, even though it's yucky and uncomfortable. Why? Because it helps us understand what our diagnosis means. It helps us to understand the impact of what's happening.

For example, with a long-term illness, that can naturally be a chronic source of anxiety. We look at it up and down, we go over and over it and we may even ruminate about it. I liken it to chewing on gristle. We're chewing and chewing and we don't want to spit it out, especially in front of others. Sometimes, if we chew on it and spend some time with it, we can actually swallow it and move past it.

So that's what we need to do. We should look around at what's going on, be okay with being uncomfortable for a bit and chew on the gristle.

RJS: What about if we're stuck with negative thoughts that don't seem to give us a break?

DAB: Coping skills can help us give ourselves grace. Instead of beating yourself up and saying, "Ugh, I'm having those bad thoughts again," and feeling worthless, you exercise some kindness in your own direction. You're as gentle with yourself as you would be with a loved one. You ask, "What do I need right now?"

And you make a list of coping skills and activities to have ready when you need them. Some examples would be walking, reading, listening to music, practicing deep breathing, knitting or other meditative crafts, journaling, drinking a cup of tea or calling a friend. But a coping skill or activity can really be anything that provides relief and is healthy and positive for you.

Once you have your list on paper, I suggest tucking it into a silverware drawer or in the folds of a sweater so that you'll find it unexpectedly as a reminder later. We need to continually reinforce and practice our coping skills to keep them available to us when they can be most helpful.

RJS: It's so hard to see your partner suffering, feeling weak, fainting or not being able to eat, for example. How can you cope with feelings of sadness or worry?

DAB: One of the things that is most helpful is reframing. To reframe, you first have to acknowledge what's going on in your thoughts and feelings: "My partner is not doing as well as they were, and this is hard for me. It's overwhelming. I'm scared, I'm feeling hopeless."

These are all normal emotions, but what do we want to focus on? Who do we want to be right now in the situation? Do we need to take a step away to be able to process what's going on for ourselves?

RJS: I always compartmentalized. It helped me in this situation. One time, I had to run out to the store, and while I was away for just seven minutes, Melissa fainted. I came back and found her collapsed on the floor of the foyer. I just went into emergency mode and kind of put my feelings in a box. I don't know if that was right or wrong, but when I think about it now, it was terribly stressful.

DAB: You did what you had to do in that moment. Some of us are very good at that. But sometimes we struggle with the idea of what is happening—you know, what it all truly means. "What am I supposed to take from this? Am I going to focus on the fact that I have the skills and I can handle it, or that I don't know what I'm doing and I need some help?" We have to take this information, process it and figure out the meaning behind it. This is where a therapist can help us figure out what we feel is in our best interest.

The idea is to discover what resets you, what gives you perspective. For me, for example, it's a walk. With a little fresh air and movement, I can view any situation differently. I can reframe it. Sometimes, when dealing with a chronic illness, it's tough to find an opportunity to hit the reset button, so it's even more important to know what gives us perspective so we can prioritize and use those levers when we need to.

RJS: You need that reset or you'll have two disasters, yes? When you don't think you know what to do, should you pause, process and then focus on what's next?

DAB: For some people, yes, they do look at that next step. For others, they need to stay in the moment or even to reflect on the fact that they figured out how to handle it.

But even when we feel we haven't handled a difficulty well, we have to give ourselves grace. With a chronic or extended illness, it's all about the long term, and the goal posts will move.

RJS: What about sleeping problems?

DAB: The purpose of sleep is to regenerate, repair. When we can't sleep, we're so anxious that our brain isn't shutting down. We'll be impacted by that, because that regeneration is blocked. If you've had sleep issues, you can get stuck on the same thoughts over and over, and this just creates restlessness and prevents actual rest.

If you have trouble falling asleep, one helpful tool is to develop a sleep routine. This can be just a half hour, or as long as you need to prepare for rest. It sounds obvious, but in our busy and largely digital lives, it's not so easy and requires thoughtful planning.

What do I need to send my brain the message that it's time to sleep? For me, taking a warm shower is a kind of symbol. A shower lets me imagine all my stressors falling off me and whirling down the drain. With that burden lifted, I can focus on being thankful and prioritizing my rest so I can be the person I want to be tomorrow. I tell myself, "You did everything you could do today, and now you get to rest and restore so you can greet the new day as you'd like."

RJS: Normally I shower in the morning, but during the last two years of Melissa's illness, I also showered at night. It was just as you said, a cleansing feeling. It really helped.

DAB: We have to change our patterns. We're all different, but we all need to understand how to start winding down. Maybe that also includes journaling about gratitude and things that happened during the day.

RJS: And what about anger? What if you're just really mad that this is all happening to you and your family or partner? How can you manage that?

DAB: Again, I'd suggest using your list of coping skills, and I'd call out journaling especially because it can really be a release to get things down on the page. You don't have to pressure yourself to write a lot—even one sentence can be helpful.

If you wake up with a difficult thought, tell yourself you already recorded it earlier in the journal. At night, if I feel stressed, I ask myself to revisit a place that is calming—the beach or the mountains, for example. Then, I check in with all my senses. What do I see, what do I hear? Waves, birds, smells? Feel the sand, feel the touch. This active observation is meditative and soothing, and you can always repeat the activity or choose another setting to visit in your imagination.

RJS: Many people have to play the role of caregiver at home and then still keep up with work, an office and other obligations. At work, should you keep difficult feelings to yourself and compartmentalize them or be open about them with your colleagues, for example?

DAB: It's not healthy to always compartmentalize. At times, yes, but at work, there's a chance you might be triggered by a remark or a situation, so you need to be certain you know who your people are.

As to choosing what to say, what are your goals in regard to talking about the illness? If you share details with someone and you know they'll keep it confidential and that's what you want, great.

If you talk to someone who isn't great at keeping things confidential, you'll want to proceed with caution. Who are the people I want in my inner circle at work? Then, beyond sharing and just in general, some days we have to acknowledge that work is not working. A serious medical battle disturbs equilibrium and can mess with focus and productivity. There are times when you're just not in the right space, and that's normal. You may need to take some time. Maybe you just sit in your car and activate one of your coping skills for a few minutes, or maybe you need to take the day to recalibrate yourself.

One other important note is, as you mention earlier in the book, the Family and Medical Leave Act is a resource for you if you or your partner are employed by a company that's covered. Make sure to speak with your HR team, because you can take unpaid time off and there is quite a bit of flexibility. You should learn your rights and use what you need to take care of yourself.

RJS: How can you deal with setbacks or disappointing or frustrating news from your medical team? The way I coped was just taking the problem and breaking it down, where I'd say, "This is what we have to do, and this is the procedure." Getting organized, putting it into a plan and then executing. Strategy, organize, execute. I realize that's coming from my entrepreneurial approach to almost everything, but you know what? It worked.

DAB: I think the important thing here is that we are all different. That organized and proactive approach worked for you, and it helped you because it was a familiar coping tool.

Then, on the complete opposite end of the spectrum, I had a client who liked to put all her cards on the table in our sessions. She'd swear, cry and scream about how unfair life was. And then, after some minutes, she'd take a deep breath, wipe her eyes and say, "It's time for me to put my big girl panties on." She needed to acknowledge the feelings, to let them flow through and out, to process them and then move forward.

RJS: Sometimes, we'd talk to other people, and I remember they'd be sharing about a crisis in their life, something they perceived as really serious, and I'd just be thinking, "How is that little thing a crisis?" Compared to what Melissa and I were going through, most other problems of daily life seemed so small. Why is it that for some people there is a much more dramatic reaction to hardship?

DAB: Well, it's not about that one thing that sets them off. It's the hundred things that came before that set the stage for a reaction of, "I just can't deal with it."

The more you get to know yourself, the more you can figure out techniques that work for you. We all struggle with something. We internalize a lot of negative messages. But we are each who we need to be right now. So, let's figure out what you need to be able to handle the situation. That's important for any couple as well, in terms of how partners relate to each other. As an example, I've worked with couples where one partner is what I call a "fixer." They just love to solve other people's problems.

RJS: Ha! Melissa always said that about me, even before she was sick. What can I say? It's my nature to fix things. I think it's a problem for me. Melissa would always accuse me of being an expert, and I would always want to solve issues. She said, "Well, that might work for you, but not for everyone."

DAB: Well, I know it comes from a place of love, but often when we're in crisis or even just dealing with something challenging, we don't actually want someone to fix it for us. We just want you to listen and acknowledge what we've said.

I think you can say, "Okay, it's in my nature to do that, but I'm going to work on just listening and acknowledging what my partner has told me."

Some people also think that with therapy, it's about getting a therapist to "fix you," but that's not it at all. Therapy is an opportunity to make a connection and to start learning how to figure things out yourself while not feeling alone.

I'm always honored and humbled to be on that journey with each of my clients, and when I see them building their toolkit of coping skills and using them in a way that is kind to themselves and true to the person they want to be, I feel really grateful to have been a part of it.

A COPING SKILLS RECAP FROM DR. ALISE BARTLEY

Coping is something we all do, whether we are aware of it or not. Some coping skills build strength and resilience, while others are a distraction. It's important to keep in mind that any coping skill you rely on should have positive consequences, not negative ones. The following is a potential list of positive coping skills. Remember: Your personal list is for you, so you are only limited by your own needs and creativity.

Diversion Coping

- Take a walk
- Write
- Sing
- Dance
- Draw
- Color
- Garden
- Go for a drive
- Watch television or a movie
- Watch cute videos on YouTube
- Read

Social/Interpersonal Coping

- Spend time with family or friends

- Talk to someone you trust
- Text or write a note to someone you care about
- Serve someone in need
- Spend time with your pet
- Encourage others

Cognitive Coping

- Write a list of pros and cons for decisions
- Make a gratitude list
- Place an inspiration quote on your bathroom mirror
- Write a list of goals
- Reframe negative feelings to positive ones
- Reward or pamper yourself when successful
- Write a list of strengths
- Accept a challenge with a positive attitude

Physical Coping

- Take a shower or a bath
- Eat healthy foods
- Rest
- Get enough sleep
- Get into a good routine
- Limit caffeine
- Limit alcohol
- Practice slow, deep breathing

CHAPTER TAKEAWAYS:

- Prioritize your connection with your partner and work on it actively
- Tell your partner you love them every single day
- Respect your partner's boundaries
- Stay in the now as much as possible
- If it's less than a seven, let it go
- Develop a set of coping skills so you'll be ready when you need them

"THE HUMAN CAPACITY FOR BURDEN IS LIKE BAMBOO— IT'S FAR MORE FLEXIBLE THAN YOU'D EVER BELIEVE AT FIRST GLANCE."

—Jodi Picoult

We Were Better Together

Chapter 6
LET LOVE FUEL YOUR JOURNEY

Hunbun,

Do you remember talking about how maybe we hadn't appreciated our love enough before the cancer? It had always been easy with us, so maybe we just didn't give it a lot of thought.

I don't say that it was "easy" to be dismissive or to sound proud. It's not that we never disagreed, and we both always had strong opinions. But the fact is, nothing really ever came between us. Being together was always comfortable and fun. We knew each other so well, we didn't sweat the small stuff and we gave each other the respect and support to pursue our goals and passions, many of which were happily shared.

Years into our battle against this disease, we agreed that our love had truly deepened in ways we couldn't have anticipated. With all my heart and soul, I loved caring for you, and I was surprised at

how naturally it came—all in spite of me originally thinking I wouldn't be a good caregiver, that I wouldn't be able to handle all that it demanded and implied.

I can't say I'm thankful for the cancer that took you from me, but I will always be grateful for the way we loved each other through it.

Bob

PRACTICAL ADVICE

Melissa had such a sweet and tender way of sharing her love and appreciation, even when she was too ill to show me in all the "normal" ways. There were times when I worried that I wasn't skilled enough at caring for her, that I couldn't do enough. Yet she spoke to me so gently. We held each other close, knowing that we had created a bond forged out of a love that was already strong, but became so much more enduring and profound through the level of true intimacy that this experience required of us.

Along the way, we learned a lot about what love really is, and what being intimate really meant, so I'm dedicating this chapter to sharing what we discovered and what worked for us. You should, as always, learn and celebrate what works for you.

Intimacy Isn't Just Sex

Make space and time to nurture your emotional intimacy and your true connection with your partner. That means different things to each couple, but it could involve quiet conversation, a warm smile, offering to listen or asking, "What do you need right now?"

Commit to Ongoing Conversation about Your Pleasure and Needs

This is especially important when it comes to physical expressions of your love, and whether you are the caregiver or the patient. Be kind but honest, and if you can, try to establish this line of communication very early on. Even if you feel a little nervous to ask questions or say what you want or need, it can really be worth it in terms of understanding and deepening your bond.

Make an agreement to listen to each other and to remain respectful and open to things that may need to change. You might even want to speak that out loud as a kind of vow, saying something like, "I will always listen and stay open to your needs, and we'll honor each other's changing desires."

To Nurture Sexual Intimacy, Be Willing to Take Things a Little Slower

Whatever your former patterns, an illness brings transformation. Often, the reality of facing an illness together opens the space for a more profound connection, even sexually. Changing routines, trying alternatives and discovering what works for you as a couple right now may take time. Be flexible, experiment and maybe go at a more leisurely pace with less pressure so you both can benefit from shared and deepening intimacy.

Limit Outside Influences That Can Inhibit Sexual Function and Reduce Pleasure

For example, if you normally have sex at night after a big meal, you might want to consider shifting your sexual schedule to avoid times when your body is fatigued or busy digesting food.

It's true, too, that alcohol decreases blood flow to the penis. Sure, a glass of wine can help us relax, but too much may create difficulty for men, specifically in getting or maintaining an erection. During a long-term illness such as cancer, you may want to limit anything that could put additional obstacles between you and potential intimacy with your partner.

Don't Be Afraid to Use a Little Help

Though you may already use some aids in your sexual life, some women can experience additional vaginal dryness, for example, as a result of treatment. In these situations, remembering to add a water-based lubricant (or use more than usual) can be very helpful to prevent pain. You might also explore using toys to help with arousal, for example.

Anticipate Small Sensory Changes That May Affect Being "In the Mood"

As just one example, some patients find that chemotherapy or other drugs can leave a metallic taste in their mouth, which can make them not want to kiss their partners. To help with this, keep mints on hand or buy a new toothbrush to help you feel fresh, and pay attention to other small ways to make intimacy easier.

Be Flexible and Hold Space for the Sweetness in Your Relationship

Cancer, or any long-term illness, can cast a shadow over everything else in our lives. Don't let that happen. Protect and nurture your time together, laugh with one another and find ways to let your love flourish even in this challenging time.

HELP FROM THE EXPERTS

I've said it before, but I can't overstate how much closer Melissa and I became as a result of her getting cancer. I never would've predicted that in the "before times," but the challenges we faced both forced and encouraged us to open up our hearts in new ways, and to be at once stronger and more vulnerable to and for each other.

Like any couple dealing with an illness, we had to have serious and deep discussions, but we also prioritized having fun, laughing and appreciating each other out loud. A lot of people probably think that intimacy and illness don't go together, but that's not true at all. We chose to see the situation as an opportunity to love and trust even more deeply and truly, and that's what intimacy meant for us.

In that same vein, all of the smart insights in the following conversation with Dr. Alise Bartley are things every couple can use to help maintain and deepen their shared connection—not in spite of the challenge of illness, but because of it.

MAINTAINING INTIMACY DURING A MEDICAL CRISIS: A Frank and Important Conversation with Dr. Alise Bartley

Robert J. Shearer: Can you help us understand the difference between physical and emotional intimacy in a committed romantic relationship?

Dr. Alise Bartley: Physical intimacy is defined as any kind of physical touch, such as holding hands, caressing, hugging or having sexual intercourse. Emotional intimacy is so much more complex. It's a connection between two people who can share freely without judgment, who can activate that connection sometimes even without talking. It also has its roots in trust and dependability. If I'm vulnerable, can I share that with my partner? Will they respond in a way that meets my needs?

RJS: What are some of the ways that love and intimacy are tested during a medical crisis such as cancer?

DAB: This is a big question. It partly has to do with our bodies not being able to respond in all the ways we used to. Our functioning changes, whether as a result of the illness, our medication or other factors related to treatment. This can obviously have an impact on our sexual, emotional and physical intimacy, and it's something that every couple needs to address individually.

RJS: When it comes to sex, sometimes medications, treatments and the disease itself can create obstacles to a fulfilling experience. Do you have any tips for couples navigating a long medical battle that is impinging on their sex life?

DAB: Yes, and this is really important to understand. For some of us, our arousal has changed. For men, it can be difficult getting or maintaining an erection or reaching orgasm. For women, it's important to remember that the vagina is a muscle. If a woman has had a round of chemo and is now feeling better, she may still sense that, sexually, things aren't working exactly as before. There may be problems with pain or even dryness, for example. Most importantly, there may be additional patience required of both partners as they figure out what works and what feels really good.

When dealing with intimacy, it's mainly about communication. Talk to your partner. Ask questions. Can we actually have sex in the traditional sense where we are right now in the illness? If not, what can we do to maintain our closeness in that way?

Bob, to your point, I absolutely encourage everyone to talk with their doctor about any and all medications and to ask specifically if there are possible sexual side effects. This is really, really important, because you may think that difficulties are being caused by "you" when they're simply a biological effect of a particular medicine.

RJS: I had a friend who was going through prostate cancer treatment. He very honestly shared with me that, you know, there are different ways of satisfying your partner and getting satisfaction. For Melissa and I, even when we couldn't be intimate in a more traditional way, Melissa absolutely loved the foot massages I gave her, especially with essential aromatherapy oils.

DAB: Well, here's an interesting fact—the nerve endings in our genitals are the same as in the bottom of our feet! But it really depends on where physical touch is in your own love language. How important is touch to you? The couple needs to take a step back and say, "If we can't physically have sex right now, how can we incorporate and embrace alternatives that are satisfying? How can we delight our senses, find ways to be creative, show our love, and enjoy each other's bodies?"

One great tool is to activate the senses. Using scents—like aromatherapy oils, as you mentioned, or fresh flowers—or playing soft music to create atmosphere and the like.

RJS: You know, one really helpful thing for us was at our first important pre-surgery appointment, the doctor was just fantastic in explaining to us how long we had to wait to have sex again after the hysterectomy. She kind of opened up the conversation for us, which made it easier. But aside from discussing it with their medical provider, how can a couple talk about intimacy and their individual needs or desires in an open and honest way that is productive but also kind?

DAB: During a serious illness, as the patient, we know our body has changed. As the caregiver, our needs may be very different—we might still be wanting more when it's just not possible. We need to pay attention to that truth and communicate with our partner.

You know, just talk about it. "What can we do? Could we change positions or make other adjustments?" Keep the conversation flowing. Be honest, but offer ideas that still preserve your closeness, that beautiful exchange that is just for you two. You could say something like, "Right now, I'm honestly not in the right place. Could we just hold each other and caress each other?" This might involve touching the erogenous zones or not—whatever works for you. The main thing is that even though function has changed, it's still a moment of shared pleasure, and it's a celebration of your love.

RJS: Just personally as the caregiver, I think it's kind of unkind to focus too much on yourself when it comes to your sexual needs when your partner is fighting for his or her life. For me, it was always about when Melissa was in the mood: "You tell me."

Then again, maybe that's related to age. Putting your own needs aside is probably easier when you're in your 60s or 70s as I was, while it might be more difficult for a younger partner. Are there sacrifices that need to be made with regard to love and intimacy during a long medical crisis?

DAB: It's about understanding what each member of the couple needs. If the cancer patient can't have sex and their partner has a more powerful sex drive, they might reluctantly choose to go outside the marriage to meet their needs. This is why you have to have an understanding and a clear agreement, or else it can be another barrier in the relationship.

Bob, for you, it didn't cross your mind—but for others, it may mean something different, and it may not be a reflection of diminished love. But if one partner seeks outside satisfaction secretly, this can definitely damage the relationship. Even if you think you won't hurt your partner, they will likely be able to tell, especially if you've been together for a long time.

The bottom line: Whatever arrangement you make, and especially if it involves changing important aspects of your intimacy, you need to talk about expectations and consequences. It's all about clarity. I often have to work through this with clients and direct the conversation so that they can think about what it all means long-term. They need to figure out how it all fits within their relationship and what the consequences are. Sometimes the person who is ill gives permission, but what is the structure of that permission?

These are not easy questions. Therapy can really help in these cases, because someone else can open these conversations and questions objectively, giving room for both people to share their thoughts in a safe space.

CHAPTER TAKEAWAYS:

- Intimacy is so much more than sex
- Communicating clearly and with compassion is key
- Be flexible and understand that you may need to take things slower
- Don't be afraid to ask your healthcare team about how medications and treatments may affect your sexual health and desire
- Find new ways to share pleasure and eliminate elements that can hamper closeness

"OUR MOST IMPORTANT SEXUAL ORGAN IS NOT BETWEEN OUR LEGS. IT'S BETWEEN OUR EARS."

—Unknown

Chapter 7
THE LONG AND WINDING ROAD

My Sweetest Love,

Do you remember that day, about two years into your treatment, when we were in the car? You know the day I mean. We'd just been to your doctor to review your latest blood work and scans. The news wasn't good, yet we held hands and agreed to stay positive. We would focus on getting past this setback and moving forward. We would beat cancer. It would not beat us.

But then in the car, the phone rang. It was the veterinarian's office. He told us Mr. Sparks was dying. Sparky—our favorite little dog, your constant companion—had cancer, too. It was just too much. Until that moment, I hadn't seen you really break down and sob, even about your own diagnosis. We cried together, and despite our philosophy of relentless optimism, we were thrown for a loop by the news. It might've been our only "Why us?" moment, and the sadness and grief didn't subside easily.

Throughout that same week, Sparky died, you had all your beautiful hair cut off (because you knew the treatment was going to make it fall out in clumps) and you got your first wig.

It was such a low point for us, but we navigated through it—together, like always, and by using our faith and leaning on each other. I really struggled with how soon to get you another dog, but I eventually decided to go ahead and bring a new puppy home. I'll always be glad I did, because it gave you a new creature to love and care for. That was always when you were happiest, and your happiness was mine, too.

I miss you so very much.

Bob

PRACTICAL ADVICE

As you may have noticed by now, in the title and structure of this book, I've chosen the metaphor of a journey as a way of framing what it's like to "go through" cancer. This chapter, as its name implies, is centered on how slow and repetitive and sometimes even monotonous the process can feel while you're devoting most of your time to making, getting to, going through and then recovering from all of the appointments, tests, scans, conversations, decisions and, ultimately, treatments and medications. It is definitely a marathon, not a sprint.

Melissa and I spent eight years on this voyage through uncharted territory, and she was never fully in remission, so it was kind of like a never-ending road trip. We had to keep going, but we also had some good fun along the route. Sure, sometimes we broke down, but we fixed ourselves up and kept on going.

Long-term illness teaches us resilience, patience and a whole lot of other things, too. In the list that follows, I hope you'll find some shortcuts to a better experience.

In Dark Times, Try to Practice Acknowledgment without Judgment

This doesn't mean accepting defeat or throwing in the towel—quite the opposite. Meditation experts often tell those with pain or injuries to observe their pain and to notice it without judgment. That may seem easier said than done, but you can cultivate this practice, and you may find it really helpful.

Melissa and I had already been through years of treatment, ups and downs, progress and setbacks. And then, wouldn't you know it, a global pandemic came along! We took it very seriously, as it made Melissa so much more vulnerable to becoming infected, but you know what? We actually chose to laugh about the irony of it. Because it just felt better to laugh.

Throughout your own experience with long-term illness, there will inevitably be some moments that are stormy and deeply emotional and possibly difficult turns on that long road. It may feel like the wind is against you and you just can't handle it. But together, you *can* handle it. Acknowledge what has occurred, but try not to judge the situation. Reassure yourself that you're not alone. Then, gently guide your attention back to the path of self-care and proactive steps toward healing. You may find that prayer or meditation and breathing exercises can offer relief as well.

Let Go of the Idea That Everything Will Go "Back to Normal" Someday

I started this book with the idea of the before and after, and that applies even when you successfully beat cancer. Both the patient and the caregiver will be changed by this process, and that is not necessarily negative. Melissa's cancer tested me as a partner in ways I couldn't have predicted, and it brought us so much closer together as a couple.

Prepare to Be Changed as a Person

Melissa and I bought long-term care insurance well before she was ever sick. We had discussed the fact that neither one of us thought we'd be good caregivers if anything should happen to the other one, but in the end, it was absolutely the opposite. Melissa didn't want anyone else to care for her, and I found that I cherished even the very real difficulties that come with caring for someone who is very ill.

To illustrate what I mean more specifically, I'll share a very personal story. At the beginning of Melissa's treatment, I added some little comforts to our master bathroom in case she wanted to have a nice bath—really just to make her feel good. At a certain point, I added a bidet when she was feeling a bit weaker, and she really liked that. Deeper into her treatment, she was spending more time there, so I added a new, more comfortable seat to the toilet. As her disease progressed in the later years, I kept a portable toilet near our bed so that I could have it ready. And in the end, I changed her bed pads and cleaned and dressed her myself.

I remember Melissa asking me if I'd ever imagined this when we'd taken our vows.

"Well," I said, "I guess that's why they put that 'in sickness and in health' part in there." And you know what? That made her smile.

Actively Notice Life's Tiny Pleasures

Give thanks for a beautiful day, a nice meal, a silly joke, drinking coffee together, your window garden or meeting a friend in the grocery store. These tiny goodnesses go a long way to redirecting stressed minds and soothing sadness and fear.

Opt for Small Sweetnesses over Aggressive Positivity with Your Partner

While I wholeheartedly support staying relentlessly optimistic, make sure you're authentic and not too pushy with the "keep your chin up" type advice and pressure. Melissa had a strong BS detector, and she absolutely didn't want me to sugar-coat anything. But I loved to compliment her, so I would bring her little gifts (a bouquet of flowers, a scented candle), and I always made a point of noticing how beautiful her skin was or how much I liked her new short hair.

Accept That Tastes and Desires May Change During Treatment

Give your partner permission to just rest, eat things they never liked before or refuse their former favorite dishes. Be flexible when plans change because they're too tired to do whatever you had planned. Let them be who they need to be right now.

As an example, for the first four years, Melissa didn't have a lot of trouble with eating or food in general, aside from being a bit nauseous in the very beginning. She worked with her nutritionist and felt that food was helping her recovery. She tried to minimize her sugar intake, as she'd always loved sweets, but later, her tastes did change and her appetite waned. At that stage, I tried to find things she liked (a milkshake as a special treat for example), or I just followed her lead when she really didn't feel like eating.

Use Art and Creativity as a Means of Expression and Healing

Whether playing a musical instrument, listening to soothing sounds, painting with watercolors or writing poems, creativity can play an integral role in the journey of both caregiver and patient. Creative expression in all its forms offers relief and can even spark joy and hope.

If there's something you've always wanted to try, do it now. If you're not sure how to get started, stop into an arts and crafts boutique or a shop that sells musical instruments and ask for guidance.

As I've mentioned before, another great outlet for expression is journaling. You can simply pick up a notebook, or, if you want something that frames how important your thoughts are, you can find a special journal that really speaks to you. Then, write what you're feeling. Describe your day, what you're angry or sad about, what you're thankful for and anything else that surfaces. Don't judge your writing or overthink it. Just let it flow.

For the Caregiver: Again, Please Take Care of Yourself

I've mentioned this in other chapters, but it bears repeating: It takes a heroic effort to manage the care of someone who is undergoing serious medical treatment. Psychologically, sometimes I was really afraid, especially the few times Melissa fainted and I had to call an ambulance.

Here's my advice:

- **Get outside.** I woke up an hour before Melissa every day to take the dogs on a long walk. Just that bit of fresh air and connection with nature was enough to clear my head and get me ready for the day.
- **Confide in a friend.** Find someone who can listen and share your experiences with them.
- **Reach out to your faith community.** Create strong connections and accept help when it's offered.
- **Talk to a professional therapist or psychologist.** This is not simple stuff, and just having an objective listener to help you sort out your feelings can be a game changer.

HELP FROM THE EXPERTS

In looking at the name of the conversation below, you may be asking yourself, "Wait a minute—if we're in the middle of a cancer journey, why are we skipping ahead to palliative care? Isn't that for dying?"

Before Melissa's diagnosis, and even well into her treatment, I would've asked the same thing. But what I came to find out through our experience is that palliative care is often completely misunderstood and almost always underused in our society. It has a bad reputation when it should be uplifted and leveraged to make life better for those experiencing significant symptoms and complications. And it doesn't necessarily have anything to do with imminent death.

So, what is palliative care, exactly? It's a multi-pronged approach to caring for people with long-term illness to help alleviate difficult symptoms and provide comfort. There's much more about it in the following exchange, but not all palliative care is hospice care.

I was fortunate enough to meet the brilliant Dr. Cameron Muir, a caring practitioner of and champion for palliative care and all its benefits to the well-being of patients facing long-term health issues. Let's dive right in, and I hope you'll discover something about the subject that may help you one day.

PALLIATIVE CARE ALONG YOUR TREATMENT JOURNEY: The Basics and Benefits of an Underused Resource Explained by Dr. J. Cameron Muir, Palliative Care Physician and Chief Innovation Officer, National Partnership for Healthcare and Hospice Innovation

Robert J. Shearer: You are a celebrated physician in the palliative care world. How did you come to work in this field? What brought you to it?

Dr. J. Cameron Muir: There are two things that really influenced me. First, as a young teenager, I watched my beloved grandmother die of lung disease. I spent a lot of time with my grandparents, and the experience of seeing her in the sterile atmosphere of the hospital, of watching my grandfather get the news over a cold phone call that she had died alone—I didn't know it then, but it shaped my future path. It was the beginning of my thinking that people shouldn't die that way, that the experience should have more humanity and warmth.

Then much later, as I was going through medical school, in my general internal medicine training, I always had this nagging question: "What are we doing and why?"

So much of training in my day was in the hospital setting, and I saw a lot of suffering there. Once people have experienced acute complications with infections or things that are not readily fixable, it can be too late.

During my medical training, I had the privilege of working with a number of brilliant people who were pioneering issues such as bioethics and informed consent. They were asking questions, too: With regard to illness, what are the choices and options that we have as patients and as people?

As an intern, I had an important experience in the hospital that shaped my perspective. I was busy with work, but I noted that one patient was really distressed, as was his daughter. I stopped to listen to them, and in those moments, I knew I was part of something important and even sacred. I went on to study medical oncology and did a fellowship in bioethics, blending metaphysics with the hardcore science.

After that, I found a palliative medicine program in Chicago. I did a hospital and palliative care fellowship, and I've now been in the field for 30 years.

So, both my personal and professional experiences have helped create my passion for changing the experience of living with advanced illness so people can be more empowered. So they can decide what's important and can even be treated in an environment where they want to be. My grandma, and many others, didn't have that option, but thankfully, things are changing.

RJS: What an inspiring story. Now, I know that a lot of people associate palliative care with hospice, so they often think that palliative care and medicine are just for the very last stages of life. I used to believe that too, but I learned that's not necessarily the case by going through the process with Melissa. Could you give us a simple primer on what palliative care actually is, and who might benefit from it?

DJCM: Palliative medicine is an umbrella term, and its purpose is to lessen the violence of disease when cure is not necessarily possible. Palliative care is non-hospice medical and counseling support for those who have symptom- and support-related needs for a serious illness.

RJS: Why is palliative care so misunderstood by patients and their families?

DJCM: Bob, if only we had a simple answer to that. The first thing is, most people don't even understand the word. Next, palliative care is not an organized benefit; it's a vague concept they sometimes just don't "get."

Palliative care isn't about just one problem affecting one body part. It's about addressing a complex set of issues that have to do with things that, as Americans, we largely don't want to discuss. Fostering a conversation around serious illness and even the acceptance of death is still counter-culture.

RJS: It's such a shame, because Melissa and I found it so helpful, and we really wished we had taken advantage of palliative care earlier in her illness. But as you said, we just didn't really "get" it, and no one took the time to explain it to us as a part of our process. It was through my own research that I came upon the idea, and it was such a lost opportunity.

DJCM: If it's a poorly presented concept—and most present it only as an end-of-life service—it's natural that most people won't understand fully. If you offer the idea more simply as help and support, it's a lot easier. Once you experience that support and what it can do, you can't imagine living without it.

Specifically in your case, your medical team probably would have brought it up in the last week or so, "at the end." That reinforces the fact that we need to change the culture and practice. We need to do better in our medical education.

If a patient brings up hospice or palliative care, most providers will discuss it, but otherwise, it's difficult and it may not come up at all until the very end. Personally, I think educating the community directly is a very effective way to help patients and their families advocate for themselves.

I do want to mention that within the cancer community, the best centers now do include palliative care as a part of their treatment offerings. That includes nutrition, survivorship, counseling and other services. In fact, cancer has been the model in the US for palliative and hospice care.

RJS: I like the idea of framing palliative care more as "help and support," and I always tell people that it's part of making the process easier on the patient. There are so many things you can do. Melissa and I were possibly a bit more proactive and willing to try different things such as acupuncture and massage. When we finally sought help from a palliative care physician, I wished I had been on top of it sooner.

Speaking of timing, when does palliative care benefit patients most? Is there a particular moment during a long-term illness when it should be considered or prioritized? If you ask me, I think it should be mentioned right away so that it's a known resource.

DJCM: It can really be useful at any point on the continuum, especially where there are big moments. Even at diagnosis there can be pain or nausea, or there may be something that needs palliating even before the diagnosis. Also, anytime there's a flare-up in symptoms, this type of care can be so important with helping to manage symptoms and helping patients cope.

We find, for example, that people who get chemotherapy for esophageal cancer and benefit from aggressive symptom management are more likely to continue their treatment. It leads to higher completion of chemotherapy and higher survival rates. That is true palliative care: unrelated to death and more a part of the process.

There are opportunities all along the way with the progression of advanced illness, COPD, pneumonia that accompanies lung disease or in any situation where bodily functions change and fear increases.

These are all good points at which to incorporate palliative care, and it can make such a difference.

RJS: In your work as a palliative care physician, what have you found most rewarding? What has surprised you?

DJCM: Families show us so much about what really matters. I find that the longer I do this work, the more it truly teaches that well-known maxim: "Don't sweat the small stuff—and it's all small stuff." Every day, every single breath, is a gift.

When I have the privilege to work with a family, at the beginning, they're often angry and sad. But how they transform, the ways in which they ultimately express love and compassion for one another—it's extraordinary and so fulfilling to witness love in its most raw and unfiltered and surprising state.

On the other hand, it still surprises me how much we twist into pretzels to avoid talking about death. It shocks me how hard we work to protect ourselves from dealing with grief and loss.

RJS: From the patient's perspective, what is the key to having the best experience with palliative care?

DJCM: Bob, you've already role-modeled that. Just ask and advocate for it, and the earlier in the process, the better.

My colleagues and I share a unified passion: We are committed to bettering the human experience, and it's our mission to make it more whole, more peace-filled. To foster the expression of love. To us, the best the patient can do is advocate for themselves or a loved one for palliative care.

RJS: What do you wish people knew that might help them take advantage of the benefits of palliative care earlier in their illness?

DJCM: That once they experience the benefits of palliative care at any point in their illness, they will without a doubt find it a crucial part of their treatment.

RJS: Yes, I'd add to that from my own experience that palliative care is the remedy that will make their journey so much easier. It's like the comfort blanket you hold when you're down and out.

Thank you so much for this conversation. Before we wrap up, is there anything else you'd like to share?

DJCM: I would reiterate the importance of advocacy for our loved ones, for ourselves and for others. It's the key to creating the best possible experience. It's what you did for Melissa, and it's what you're doing now to help those going through their own journeys.

I'd also say that honoring, remembering and creating legacy for those who have transformed our lives is a beautiful thing. Your passion for empowering others and paying tribute to Melissa through this project is an example of that.

CHAPTER TAKEAWAYS:

- Cancer and other serious illnesses are long journeys and require strategic thinking
- Meditation and other daily practices can help manage stress
- Things will not go back to "normal", as you have a new normal now
- When challenges loom large, celebrate the small victories and pleasures
- Palliative care offers great benefits even before the end-stages of disease, including helping patients have better treatment outcomes

**"WHEN YOU GET TO
THE END OF YOUR ROPE,
TIE A KNOT AND HANG ON."**

—Theodore Roosevelt

Chapter 8
THE GOOD NEWS AND WHAT'S NEXT

My beautiful Melissa,

Do you remember the times we got really good news? When the scans were clear and the blood markers were trending in the right direction? How happy we were leaving the doctor's office and stopping for lunch and making plans! It seems funny now to think that blood test results could spark total euphoria, but, well, when they were good, there was nothing that could compare.

It just felt so damn great to have our positive approach to your healing reflected back to us in real results. We were getting through this. We were triumphant, if humbly so, and your eyes sparkled.

What meant most to me about those moments was that we'd done them together, and we did that for eight years. I mean, I know it was you on the front lines, living with the illness in your own body. It was always more you than me. Still, we worked as a team on every aspect, loving and encouraging each other, doing what we had to do even when it wasn't easy and staying true to our values of determined optimism and daily gratitude. What do the kids say on social media? #couplegoals

And then, on those days when we'd been really encouraged by the doctors, we sometimes cried a little from happiness and held each other, full of hope.

Something wonderful happened to me every day for more than 30 years, and I give thanks for it even now. You loved me, my darling, and there is no better news than that.

Bob

PRACTICAL ADVICE

As I mentioned in the last chapter, Melissa was never fully in remission from her cancer. But we did have breaks where things were quiet for a month or so between scans or appointments. That being said, regardless of whether we were facing good or bad news, we had a daily ritual.

Every night in bed, we'd make a list. Each of us would say something good that happened that day, and often it was a detail so small we might never have noticed it in the before times. We'd seen a cute movie, talked to friends or had fun with the dogs. But those things, and the gratitude we offered for them, meant so much.

For those who have received the happy news of improvement from a great scan as well as those looking at remission or even becoming "cancer-free," there is clearly so much relief and joy. But there can also be a looming sense of uncertainty, of waiting for something else to happen, of not knowing what to do now that there is hopeful news. I wanted this chapter to address how good news can impact your way forward, so let's dive right into some strategies for navigating what's next.

First and Foremost, Do Celebrate Any and All Good News

Good news may be a good ultrasound, improved blood work or an increase in weight. It could also be that moment when you're declared "cancer-free." Whatever the positive development, take the time to acknowledge your progress and be grateful for it.

I just can't say enough about how important and restorative gratitude was for us in our process. The very act of giving thanks brought relief, comfort and a sense of peace. Sometimes, when we're "fighting a battle," as many of us refer to the existential struggle with cancer, we just put our heads down and ready ourselves for the next bit of bad news. I suggest that you refuse to live that way, and that you always look for what can be celebrated, large or small.

To be clear, I'm not suggesting you live in denial of facts or that you mask your true feelings—not at all. I'm merely saying that for Melissa and me, when we were able to shift our energy toward thankfulness, it lifted our moods, made our challenges more manageable and, frankly, kept the joy and happiness of our life where it needed to be: front and center.

Continue Seeking Support Where You Need It

If you're fortunate enough to have come through cancer and are in remission or have been declared "cancer-free," you may expect yourself to just bounce back into life as individuals and as a couple. Back to work, back to routines—and that's all good.

But remember that you may still need extra emotional support to help you transition, and that transition may be bumpy. That's normal. Just because the physical manifestations of the illness are gone, that doesn't mean that the healing is complete. And if you are feeling a looming fear that your disease will come back or experiencing inertia or other uncomfortable sensations when you think about what to do next, that's normal, too. Don't be afraid to prioritize yourself. My suggestion is to opt for extra support, even when the news is good.

Stop Holding Your Breath

Clearly, this is easier said than done, especially because, after months or even years of treatment and a successful outcome, it's only natural to worry that the disease will return. But with support and time, you can move forward into a new phase of life, one where you'll hopefully have an enhanced appreciation of what really matters and what you want for yourself and your life together.

You'll have the benefit of having come through something so difficult, and that kind of struggle can bring with it an enormous amount of clarity. Take advantage of that, and allow yourself the freedom to breathe and to move forward.

Use the Good News to Help You with Important Planning

If there are things you'd like to organize or address but have been putting off while dealing with treatment, now may be a good time to look at those. I'm talking about tasks such as estate planning, getting documents together and that sort of stuff—not anyone's favorite project, but taking advantage of good news can give you more strength and resilience as you deal with things that might normally feel more difficult or annoying. Plus, having all your ducks in a row, even when you're now healthy and happy, can bring you a sense of pride and comfort in knowing that you did what you needed to do.

Try "Square Breathing"

Also known as "Box Breathing," Dr. Alise Bartley suggests this technique for those who don't generally enjoy meditating but still want the relief and benefits that focused breathing can bring.

It's simple and easy to do no matter where you are. If you like, you can also choose a word or "intention" to focus on, such as "healing" or "calm" or whatever works for you. Some people like to picture the breath traveling around a square shape, but most important is just to focus on your breath and the count.

1. Sit with your back supported and close your eyes.
2. Inhale slowly for a count of 4 (1,2,3,4).
3. Hold your breath for a count of 4.
4. Slowly exhale for a count of 4.
5. If you have time, repeat one or two more cycles.

HELP FROM THE EXPERTS

As it relates to a serious health challenge, good news is, well, *great.* But how we deal with positive developments and good news—how we view them, and how we fold that new reality into our lives—is a very individual practice that can benefit from thoughtful attention. Good news can bring its own set of stressors and anxieties, but it's also an opportunity to move forward.

Below are two conversations that are so important when you're transitioning through good news in your health journey. The first is another enlightening and advice-filled interview with Dr. Alise Bartley, where she offers strategies for dealing with good news in whatever form it takes for you—with advice not only on how to keep living but to actually thrive.

The second is an exchange with estate planning expert Andrew Krause. This may seem odd for a "good news" chapter, but if you've read the bullet points above, you'll understand my logic. Estate planning is so important, even if you don't think you've got much to organize. Just having your documents and wishes in order will help your loved ones so much in the future, and you can take advantage of moments when you're not so bogged down in treatment to really get organized. I hope you'll find the advice helpful and motivating.

MOVING ON FROM CANCER: Dr. Alise Bartley on Addressing the Complex Feelings That Can Accompany Even the Good News

Robert J. Shearer: When Melissa and I got good news, it was always exciting, but we still lived with a sense of doubt, in three-month increments between her scans and blood work. How do you cope with the real sense of uncertainty that comes after "winning" a battle with cancer? How do you deal with that on a daily basis?

Dr. Alise Bartley: For months or years, cancer has been in front of your face. It's been your focus. Now, maybe it's in remission, so it's off to the side. But speaking honestly, the furthest it will likely ever be is in your peripheral vision.

Now, you need to decide: Do I want to continue to focus my gaze on the cancer, on the disease, or to make a shift back toward living my life? You can choose to take everything that goes with the cancer—envisioning and acknowledging it—and then set it aside. It's still there, but you're setting it aside. Also, ask yourself: What lessons do I want to take from this? We all have to process the meaning of each stage of our medical journey. How do we want to frame it? We have the power and the right to place it in a space that is as comfortable as possible.

You can say, "I know I had cancer, but I'm going to set it at 70 degrees, and I'm not going to focus on it. I'm going to focus on sleeping well, eating well and getting my scans so that I have power and control." Everything you know about who you are has shifted. When you make a decision to set it aside, you take your power back. I'm not suggesting to shut it off or completely compartmentalize it. Acknowledge it, and then move forward.

RJS: How do you set long-term goals again after having been singularly focused on fighting something that was trying to kill you?

DAB: Time helps. The further we are from the experience, the more opportunity we have to separate from it. That passage of time will help, but what we can do as that time is passing is decide how we will use our time.

One phase I talk about is *detachment*. During detachment, we have apathy: "I don't care," "I won't care" and even "I can't care." But we become very introspective, which is good: "What does this all mean to me?" When you're told you're in remission, you need to be introspective, and ask, "What do I want to do with all this?"

Then, we move to a stage of *reorganization*. I prefer to focus more on reorganization rather than on acceptance. For me, it's more about the idea that we can *reorganize*. It's an inner peace, renewed involvement, new insights, optimism and joy. A retaking of your own power and setting new goals. You have to allow this to change your life, but you can redefine what that means. You don't have to be the person with cancer. You can choose who you are in your story. Survive, thrive—whatever works for you.

RJS: Can you say more about the importance of feelings in general throughout this process?

DAB: We are made of thoughts, behaviors and feelings. We are *made of them*. The body gives us information about our feelings—when we get those sweaty palms or our heart beats faster or we're nauseous or have trouble sleeping or breathing.

I strongly encourage you to actually acknowledge your feelings. This step is crucial before moving on. We don't have to judge our feelings —they're all valid. We don't have to say sorry for crying. After all, would you ever apologize for laughing at something funny?

Feelings deserve all your respect and acknowledgment that they are rooted in the intensity of what life really means. They are an expression of the meaning in our lives.

THE BASICS OF ESTATE PLANNING: The When, What, Why and How of Estate Planning to Benefit Your Loved Ones with Andrew Krause, Veteran Wealth Management Attorney

Robert J. Shearer: Andy, I'm so happy to be speaking with you about such an important topic. Tell us a bit about yourself and how you came to choose this type of work.

Andrew Krause: I was actually encouraged by my father to become a tax lawyer, and I took his advice. For two years during law school, I clerked for an estate planning professor. He recognized my passion and suggested I look into a Master of Law degree, which I did.

Now, having practiced for more than 40 years in the field of estate planning, tax, wealth transfer planning and estate and trust settlement, I consider myself very fortunate to have an endless passion for my work.

RJS: How would you describe your approach to estate planning?

AK: It can range from a more basic approach to a very customized, client-centric, objective-oriented service designed to address every detail.

Over the years, I've learned to ask my clients a few very important questions regarding their preferences, their beneficiaries and how the estate plan will be received. The questions mostly address what is important to the client—their relationships, the message they want to send and what type of control or access they intend for the assets they will pass along.

It's really important that you look at your own situation to come up with the plan that's right for you. A good lawyer can help you do that, and they'll take care of the necessary legal actions to make sure your wishes are carried out, whether that's through your will or a trust, for example.

RJS: Having been through this myself, I realize now how many topics can get overlooked. I mean, the obvious parts of a plan would be what you've said above, and everyone thinks of cars, homes, bank and retirement accounts. But now, we have so many digital accounts, smartphones and even social media accounts that need to be managed or deactivated. Those processes after a death can be really frustrating, so I'd imagine it's always best to plan in advance, yes? And then there are our final wishes for a funeral or celebration of life.

But many people in the US don't have a plan, even though they know they should. When you find yourself overwhelmed by a medical crisis, how can you also deal with "getting organized" to create an end of life/estate strategy?

AK: I can't say this enough: It's so much better to plan now. First off, I really encourage everybody to have the basic documents in place to empower loved ones to act on your behalf while you are still living, without court involvement to the extent possible. Then, you can put together your will and any necessary trusts or other elements based on your situation. Start now, wherever you are, and enlist the help of a good attorney, if you can. They will guide you and take some of the stress off your shoulders during a difficult time.

RJS: If you had to prioritize which documents are most important to an estate plan, what would they be?

AK: I'd recommend a durable power of attorney for financial matters, a durable power of attorney for health care decision-making, often including a health care surrogate designation, and a living will. These documents empower others to make decisions for you when you cannot make them yourself.

Also important but often overlooked is a HIPAA authorization form to enable your group of loved ones to learn about your medical condition, treatment and history from doctors, hospital workers and others in possession of your protected health information.

Some states have statutory forms for these basic documents. Just search your state government website, google "living will Ohio," for example, or ask your legal team for help.

Another important tip: If you have homes in more than one state, you will want to be sure you have documents for them that will work in each location.

RJS: Okay, and what are some next steps in the process?

AK: If you have a financial planner, they can be very helpful in organizing your financial information for presentation to your attorney so they can prepare an estate plan, whether that's just a will, a will and revocable trust or more. Lawyers typically have questionnaires which you can complete in advance.

If you don't have a financial planner, then simply giving your estate planning lawyer a list of assets, estimated values and how they're titled, along with beneficiary designations in place for IRAs and other accounts, is a good place to start.

You may be surprised to know there are laws in every state that create a default will for you if you don't make one for yourself, so it's very important to put in writing the names of individuals and/or charities you want to benefit at your death and to indicate specific amounts or percentage shares for your lawyer to reflect in your will or trust.

Also: Who should be responsible for carrying out your wishes? This will be the person working with the lawyer and other professionals who will help settle the estate. Choosing this person is really important, and you should ask them first whether they're willing to take on that role, as it can be a lot of responsibility.

RJS: Is it expensive to plan your estate? Are there options for those who may not be able to hire a legal team? In our Reading Room section at the end of the book, we've listed some resources that may be helpful to those starting to get organized, such as a Farewelling Worksheet that takes people through the process of gathering information and thinking about important questions in preparation for starting their plans.

AK: Yes, that's a really important step. And yes, unfortunately, it can be expensive to have a customized estate plan, because it takes a detailed approach and more time. But it can be argued that you or your heirs may face far greater costs if your estate plan is not efficient, optimized and organized.

That being said, there are some law schools that offer clinics where law students help clients create their plans. You can google the terms "elder clinic" and your city name, for example.

And there are lawyers who specialize in elder law, so if there aren't tax matters to deal with, presumably, that way can be less expensive. There are also online platforms that offer very basic will services, but I am not a big fan, for a variety of reasons.

RJS: Ah yes, you're talking about FreeWill and Trust & Will?

AK: Yes, among others. Of course, it depends on your circumstances and your budget, but in my opinion, online estate planning services are not as reliable at accomplishing your objectives. Often, these services don't even provide legal guidance. So although it's more expensive, you may be better off using a lawyer, even one with a simple, more standardized offering.

RJS: How can people get started in a way that will make it less stressful and overwhelming?

AK: The best way to get started is to hire a lawyer if you can, perhaps with the initial guidance of a trusted financial advisor, your CPA or a money manager. If you want to start by gathering a list of your assets, accounts and beneficiaries, that can help you when you do meet with a professional.

RJS: Is there any other advice you'd like to share for families navigating a serious illness with regard to getting things in order?

AK: If you do already have a plan when you're faced with a terminal illness, it's important to let your estate planning lawyer know, since there may be tax planning steps to consider.

A terminally ill client's estate planning lawyer, financial planner and tax advisor can review the facts and make suggestions that may result in significant tax savings for the client or their beneficiaries, possibly including estate and income taxes. Last-minute steps can sometimes be very helpful and effective.

RJS: Thanks so much for all this, Andy. I think the biggest takeaway is to start now, wherever you are, to research what type of help you might need, and then to find the right help based on your personal circumstances.

AK: Well said, and thank you. I hope this will encourage everyone to take some time now to get organized. It will really be worth it, that I can promise you.

CHAPTER TAKEAWAYS:

- Celebrate all good news, small or large, and give thanks for it
- Because even good news, as it relates to illness, can mean a big shift, make sure you have extra support in place to help you with next steps
- Use the buoyancy of good news to help you address estate planning or other outstanding issues that are important to you
- Whatever your feelings are around your good news, they are valid and they deserve your respect

"IF THE ONLY PRAYER YOU EVER SAY IS 'THANK YOU,' THAT WILL BE ENOUGH."

—Eckhart Tolle

Chapter 9
RUNNING OUT OF ROAD

My True Love,

Do you remember when we realized that our winning days against cancer were behind us?

The funny thing is, I don't think we ever really did give up or surrender, even in the later stages, did we? We always thought we'd find a way, that we'd get through the next obstacle. And you know, we did just that so many times.

I remember our very good friends, Tim and Carol. Carol died suddenly, and I recall that our conversations shifted a bit. It was as if her death had opened a doorway to a room we hadn't yet noticed. You and I started talking about our reality in more detail. We made lists of the beautiful things you wanted to share with others, just in case you couldn't use them anymore—your jewelry, a favorite handbag, a pretty vase. I remember I started the conversation about burial or cremation as if I were talking about myself someday in the future, and you picked up on that and told me what you wanted.

Looking back on it, I almost wish we could've talked about it more and earlier, but I simply couldn't acknowledge that you were going to die. I couldn't imagine a world without you. We were a team. I could only think of making you comfortable, of giving you a bath, of seeing that you'd eat a little something. I could only kiss you and hold your hand and pray with you.

I know we had 30 wonderful years together, and I thank God for each and every one of them, for every single moment we shared. But if I'm being totally honest, I would've wanted at least 30 more.

Your loving husband,

Bob

PRACTICAL ADVICE

When Melissa and I started to realize that we couldn't win our battle forever despite our valiant efforts, I wouldn't say things shifted right away. But one thing I actively did was start to listen even harder.

As I said in the letter above, when our good friend Carol died, it seemed like that opened a door for more frank, but still very gentle, conversations that touched upon death. One thing I did was to listen very intently to Melissa when she did try to tell me something, and I'm so glad I did. In those conversations, she'd tell me who she wanted to talk to and what was important to her now. What is really interesting is that listening was a gift. Melissa may have appreciated it too, but in fact, it was a gift to *me*, because I knew my wife felt safe and cared for. She knew she could trust me with whatever she needed, and that I'd do my best to make it happen.

I hope you never run out of road, or at least not for a long, long time. But here's what I'd suggest if you—and May God bless and keep you so you don't have to use these any time soon.

Get as Much Support as You Need (Which Is Probably More Than You Think)

Contact your faith leader and/or your therapist. Ask your medical professionals to help you understand in more detail what might happen next so that when some of the natural aspects of the dying process begin, you won't be too frightened. Sallie Tisdale, the brilliant writer and hospice nurse, has a book called *Advice for Future Corpses and Those Who Love Them*, which I recommend. It is a beautiful guide to what happens to a dying person and how to support them with love.

Locate and Organize Practical Information

These days, we all have so many accounts, credit cards, online profiles, passwords, professional websites and government-associated information like Social Security numbers.. Print out an online checklist and make sure you know where to find the info you'll need (will, account info for all banks, insurance and investments, log-ins and passwords). Keep them in a safe, private place rather than in the patient's hospital or hospice room. Without this info, you can find yourself in an administrative feedback loop that can make the process after someone dies much, much more difficult than it already is.

Listen, and Listen Some More

Depending upon your loved one's health status, they may not feel like or be able to talk a lot. If they do have something to say, take them seriously. If they don't want to eat, don't force them. Give them permission to feel what they're feeling and to have what they need. Show them that you hear them and that you respect their needs.

Try to Talk About Final Wishes

This can seem like an impossible or overwhelming task, and it's really better to have done it earlier in the journey if you can. But if not, gently ask to open the conversation. If you feel you simply can't, you can call on your faith leader to help with this. They can frame it in a way that offers comfort and care, so that you can know what your loved one prefers and what aligns with their values. So many people have told me that they had no idea what their loved one wanted, and it bothers them to this day that they made choices about burial, cremation or other details that they're just not sure about.

Just Be There for Your Person

You don't have to know "the right thing" to say, and it's okay to cry or for them to cry. That's a natural reaction to what is happening. Susan Halpern, author of *The Etiquette of Illness*, suggests softening questions with: "Do you want to talk about...?" rather than being more direct. This gives agency to the person who is dying to decide if it's something they do want to address.

A Note to the Dying Person: Try, If You Can, to Express Your Wishes

Be it more sunlight, a playlist that you like or just complete silence or a video call to an old friend, now is the time to say what you need and to have things your way.

Sallie Tisdale, the hospice nurse and author I mentioned above, says that her own approach when the time comes will be to remain as curious as possible as long as possible, and to try to really live—or experience—the dying process as much as she can. Will that be your approach? Whatever you want, it's not selfish to ask for it.

Consider Hospice as a Resource Earlier

This may sound controversial, because in our culture, many think that talking about or acting on hospice services implies "giving up" or is "a death sentence," but upon deeper examination, hospice is a wonderful gift you can offer yourself or your partner (and there's much more on this in the Help from the Experts section of this chapter).

A good hospice facility offers a much higher quality of life than that of a hospital, with everything from art and music therapy to advanced and personalized pain management and a warm and loving community. The folks at Hospice of the Valley in Scottsdale, Arizona, who came to our home to care for Melissa, were absolute angels on

Earth. I only wish we had taken advantage of this option sooner, so that the last few months of her life could have been even more comfortable and full.

Whenever Possible, Focus on Small Pleasures

Even in the advanced stages of an illness, you and your partner can share joyful and caring moments together. Melissa experienced pretty serious neuropathy in her feet as a result of her treatment, and as I mentioned earlier, she used to love it when I would rub her feet with essential oils. I cherished the sweet intimacy of those moments, and I just loved making her feel better. In fact, in the very late stages of her illness, I found myself a little jealous when Melissa sometimes preferred her professional caregiver's massages to mine!

HELP FROM THE EXPERTS

In thinking about what kind of "advice" to offer about such a deeply personal experience, I found myself a bit lost. Who am I to tell anyone how to approach something that I myself found so difficult, something that still lives within me even after the loss of my love?

So, I turned to Father Terry once more, and he offered this moving essay about what healing means as opposed to the idea of being cured. I hope it will offer you an opportunity to think about what true healing means for you and your partner, whether you are the patient or the caregiver.

And from the bottom of my heart, I pray that you'll feel less afraid and alone as you find yourself in this new place.

HEALING YOURSELF EVEN WHEN THERE'S NO CURE: Guidance for Those Near Death from Reverend Terence Keehan (Father Terry)

Right after I came to my parish at Holy Family in 2009, the gospel on a certain Sunday was centered on one of the healing stories. I delved into the word "cure" and the word "heal." I said that healing is a more spiritual thing, and a cure is more related to the physical body.

Sometimes, when I pray for healing for a dying person, they misunderstand me because they think I'm praying that they'll be cured physically, but I'm praying for their true healing.

But what is healing? What does it mean to heal? It's about acceptance. Healing means reconciling—putting back together something that's broken. Because of an illness, you have a greater sense of urgency to reconcile with someone you may have hurt or who may have hurt you. You may feel compelled to knock things off your bucket list. But the process of healing is really about accepting and reconciling whatever you can.

In my work with so many people who are close to death, I have seen a kind of pattern that breaks down into four scenarios around those words: "heal" and "cure."

The first is, you come through the crisis, you are cured physically, you're able to heal spiritually and you move forward. You come away with a greater appreciation of life from there on out.

The second scenario is much more difficult. Here, you unfortunately don't experience a physical cure, and you don't focus your attention on your true healing, on the acceptance and reconciliation that are so important. And you die angry and sometimes very bitter.

In the third scenario, there are folks who are physically cured, so their body comes through the disease, but they're never healed spiritually. This often leaves them feeling victimized, or like they were robbed of happiness or quality of life for an extended period of time by the illness. These feelings can last for years or even forever.

And then, finally, there are those most inspiring people, the ones who never get cured, but they heal. They've learned acceptance, and they've reconciled their lives within the illness. They'll say to me, "I've lived my life, I've made my peace and I'm in a good spot." It doesn't mean they don't have feelings of sadness about dying, but in effect, they're ready for what's to come.

Whenever there is healing to be done, I encourage people to write. Writing or journaling can be a truly healing activity, if you're well enough to do it. Therapy can also make space for awareness and acceptance, as can speaking to a spiritual leader.

That reminds me: While, as faith leaders, we always would prefer to have an ongoing dialogue with the members of our community, any one of us will always welcome the opportunity to listen to you regardless, and to share with you the guidance and comfort offered by the tenets and scriptures that are the pillars of our practice. So, don't hesitate to ask to speak to a spiritual leader at whatever point you feel it might be helpful. That is a part of what we're trained to do, and what we're called to do.

Many people don't know that religious organizations of all faiths often offer visiting teams to provide comfort, companionship and, in the case of Catholicism, even Holy Communion. These visits can be such a positive experience for a person who is nearing the end of life. Ask your community if this type of personal visit might be possible.

Often, when I visit a terminally ill person and I sense a particularly difficult struggle with letting go, I say something that family members might not be ready to say. My message to the dying is, "It's okay to let go—God will catch you." If you, as their partner, can find the space to say this with love and tenderness, it may be just what they need to make their transition in peace.

CHAPTER TAKEAWAYS:

- There is no "right way" to face the experience of death and loss, and your feelings are all valid
- Try to be as present as you can and listen more than ever
- Don't worry about saying just the right thing, just be there
- If you are dying, ask for what you need and want
- If possible, try to organize important information and documents
- Remember: healing is different than being cured

"IF YOU DON'T KNOW WHAT TO SAY TO A DYING PARTNER, SAY, 'I DON'T KNOW WHAT TO SAY RIGHT NOW, BUT I'M HERE WITH YOU AND FOR YOU.' SAY, 'I'M NOT GOING ANYWHERE. WE ARE IN THIS TOGETHER.'"

—Reverend Terence Keehan

Chapter 10

THE SURPRISING GIFTS OF HOSPICE AND PALLIATIVE CARE

Sweetheart,

I'm writing to you on the first anniversary of the day you left this world. It's not an easy day for me, and I find myself revisiting so many moments we shared.

We were always together, so in my life now, something will happen, and I'll think, "I need to tell Melissa about this." And then I remember: I can't tell you anything in the same way I used to. But I often talk to you anyway, and I hope somehow you can hear me. I tell you things I think will make you laugh, or things that seem special. Sometimes, I just say silly things, but by speaking them aloud, I feel I bring you closer to me. I guess that's what these letters are for, too.

Do you remember the time last fall when I told you about Julz, one of the young horses we were training? You had chosen her sire—her mother was one of your favorites, and you nurtured and cared for this talented up-and-comer. Just a few months after you died, our Julz became the AQHA World Champion in Senior Reining. World Champion!

When I got this news, I came home, set the urn holding your ashes on the dining room table and told you all about it. It would've meant so much to you. I know it might sound silly, but to me, Julz's victory felt like a sign. I felt your presence so strongly. I could almost feel your smile.

Now, when I go out to dinner with our friends, to a tennis tournament or even when I watch a movie, it's all bittersweet, because you're not there to share those moments with me that we once loved so much. Sometimes, I feel a pang of guilt if I laugh at a joke or feel joy at seeing a beautiful sunset, but I know you wouldn't want that. You would want me to keep going. We talked about that in your last weeks, when we found the beauty and comfort of hospice care.

I'm talking about hospice and palliative care in this chapter because I know you'd want me to share how important the experience was for us in the last few weeks of your life. Even though you volunteered for years on the board of a hospice organization, neither of us really grasped how helpful it would be (and could've been earlier) in such delicate times. It's just a topic that most of us want to avoid, but I want to change that.

If we can help even one family take advantage of its benefits, we will have accomplished another thing together, my love, even if you're not here to see it. It would be the best thing I could hope for.

I love you,

Bob

PRACTICAL ADVICE

So many people feel that accepting palliative care and/or hospice is a kind of "giving up." Many think it means they're going to die immediately, and that has a lot to do with folks waiting too long to opt into hospice when it could make them so much more comfortable.

In anticipating a move to hospice, they might feel depressed, angry, anxious, defeated or resigned. Melissa and I never really approached it from a place of sadness, but we did think it meant a quickening of the timeline toward death. Even though Melissa had served on the board of a hospice organization for years, it was a step for us as it likely will be for anyone.

Before we experienced hospice care at home in Arizona, we didn't understand how fantastic it could be and how much it could reframe all that we had to go through approaching the end of life. It doesn't take away all the pain, but it can offer anyone a layer of comfort and understanding that means everything in these moments.

What the marvelous team at Valley Hospice in Arizona did for us completely changed our perspective on end-of-life care. It was a beautiful community of pure kindness, acceptance, expertise and inspiration.

Melissa and I were both bowled over at how much hospice care helped us, and so I feel really passionate about sharing all that we discovered in the hopes that it can be a gift to you, too.

Don't Be Afraid of Palliative Care

As you'll see from the conversation that follows (and from the interview with Dr. J. Cameron Muir in Chapter Seven), it's a topic that can be confusing, but palliative care can be used throughout your illness to help manage symptoms, be treated as a whole person and get connected to other resources you may need. Read on, and prepare to be surprised at how beneficial it can be and how reframing may change your personal journey.

Don't Confuse Palliative Care with End-of-Life Hospice Care

The two can be but are not always related, and this confusion often leads patients and doctors to avoid the conversation. Palliative care can be added into other long-term medical treatment for a chronic illness, and it's really just there to reduce pain and increase comfort. It's a multi-disciplinary approach that can involve a variety of treatments.

Hospice care is a resource for when further treatment is not advised or wanted. It often also involves palliative medicine (for pain management, for example), but can also involve visiting volunteers, respite care to help caregivers have time to rest and other resources.

Ask Your Medical Team Questions Early and Be Your Own Advocate

After a diagnosis, you will have discussions with your specialist to confirm your treatment plan. You'll have an opportunity to ask questions, and one of them should be about their approach to palliative care (meaning care that helps to mitigate and reduce pain and add comfort) at various way points on the path of facing a serious illness. Let your doctor know that you are aware of this resource and that you'd like to consider it where it might be most helpful.

Be Gentle with Yourself During This Transition

When making a shift into hospice care, be kind to yourself and to your partner. Make room for your feelings, even those of sadness or anger, and allow your team to help you with counseling, volunteer visits and other resources that may help you feel more connected and supported at this new crossroads.

HELP FROM THE EXPERTS

When I first met Mike Milward, I was struck immediately by his incredible kindness and his passion for the work of hospice and palliative care. The fact that he is the CEO of America's largest not-for-profit hospice network made for an immediate connection with me and my entrepreneurial side, but when I found out that he is also a long-time chaplain and funeral celebrant, I was simply bowled over by the way he has brought his own gifts to bear to help so many families over so many years through one of the most essential human experiences. Whether welcoming families into end-of-life care, providing them medical, emotional and spiritual comfort or helping them craft meaningful ceremonies to celebrate the life of a loved one, Mike has spent decades caring for families at the crossroads between life, death and grief.

In this conversation with him (and in another that follows in the next chapter around celebrating the life of a loved one), he helps us open to the healing experience that awaits us through this practice and vocation.

Here he explains what hospice really is, what some of hospice care's various roles are and how it all can work.

UNDERSTANDING PALLIATIVE CARE AND HOSPICE FOR A BETTER END-OF-LIFE EXPERIENCE: A Conversation with Former Hospice Chaplain and Funeral Celebrant Michael Milward, CEO, California Hospice Network

Robert J. Shearer: People navigating an illness can be confused by all the terminology. What exactly is the difference between palliative care and hospice?

Michael Milward: The easiest way to think about it is that all hospice is palliative care, but not all palliative care is hospice. Palliation simply means "to reduce the symptoms of, *without curing*," so it's an overall approach to helping someone be comfortable, to reduce discomfort. That may include treatment for physical symptoms as well as addressing psychological, social and spiritual needs.

But hospice itself is not related to curative interventions. When you're on hospice, the care you receive is not geared toward curing your disease, and you're opting for palliative measures instead. It's a shift in stages of the journey.

Hospice is practical, but it's also soulful. We understand that dying is so much more than a medical event. Of course, we help attend to all the practicalities, including medical supplies, durable medical equipment and the like, but the patient and family are also accompanied by a group of compassionate, kind people to walk with them through this unique human journey.

For example, a patient with an advanced illness who has not chosen hospice can absolutely have palliative care (meaning treatment to help address pain and other issues) while they're being actively treated for their disease. It's care that helps them be more comfortable in whatever ways are needed.

RJS: What can people expect from hospice?

MM: Hospice offers so many services, managed and carried out by an interdisciplinary team. The team consists of a physician, a nurse case manager, evening and weekend visit nurses, a medical social worker and even a chaplain if you request one. We provide trained volunteers at the patient's request as well. Often, the team can also include music and/or art therapy.

And then, it's really important to mention the unsung heroes of the hospice team, the home health aides. Home health aides make visits to assist with showering, grooming, changing and other physical needs, like giving the patient a shave.

Together, the team coordinates care to create a holistic experience that takes all the patient's needs into account.

RJS: What do hospice volunteers do?

MM: Hospice volunteers undergo intensive training. People who choose to become hospice volunteers are remarkable in that they want to be companions for people at the end of life.

Volunteers develop a relationship with the patient and the family, whether that's a more traditional family, a chosen family or community that is supporting the patient. Volunteers can become trusted listeners for patients and those around them.

Their other duties may include things like grocery shopping, playing cards or watching movies, or they might stay with the patient so their family can go out to get a cup of coffee or some fresh air.

It is important to note that hospice volunteers are not medical professionals, so they don't dispense medications or attend to medical care.

RJS: On that topic, can you talk more about medical care through hospice? I know it's confusing to a lot of people.

MM: As we've discussed, hospice provides an interdisciplinary team to care for the patient. We provide regular visits, but hospice does not provide caregivers who stay around the clock in a home hospice situation.

To break it down more simply, there are four levels of hospice care. First, there's home care, where your symptoms can be managed at home or in a facility as much like home as possible—an assisted-living setting, for example. Routine home care is the most common type of hospice care. It's the largest part of what we do.

Next, there's continuous care, where the patient remains at home, but the symptoms are so profound that they require extensive nursing care every day. This requires an additional level of authorization from Medicare.

A third level of care is called general inpatient care. This is for patients with symptoms that require hospitalization, or care within a hospice inpatient unit. In this case, symptoms cannot be managed at home, so the patient is transferred to a facility and managed by a round-the-clock staff.

The fourth level is called respite care, and it's something that not a lot of families know about. It's designed to help the caregivers of someone at home. Medicare will pay for you to move the patient into an assisted-living or skilled nursing facility for a maximum of one week so that the family can take a break.

RJS: Another thing that can be confusing for families is navigating insurance coverage and hospice. How can people understand the process of enrolling in hospice and what their financial responsibility will be versus that of their health or long-term care insurance?

MM: As it relates to palliative care, hospice is a bit different. You can be on a palliative program and still be treated for your disease, curatively. We call this concurrent care. But when you choose hospice care, Medicare regulations require that you forgo curative care because it relates to the expenses of the programs. You sign a document to elect hospice care, and then Medicare pays for hospice instead of the curative treatments. Also, just as an important exception to the Medicare rules, pediatric hospice patients under 18 years old are permitted to continue seeking curative care.

Understanding how it's paid is actually very simple: Ninety-five percent of hospice recipients receive their benefit through Medicare. It's not through private insurance. It's basically free to the beneficiary —no deductibles, no loopholes. Your healthcare professional should be able to refer you.

But making a choice of the right provider is more difficult, because not all hospice organizations are created equal. There can be fraud and profiteering, and you may have more or fewer visits per week. If you're under 65 years old and don't have Medicare, most not-for-profit hospices will take everyone.

People mistakenly think hospice is one big operation, but that's not true at all. There are for-profit and not-for-profit hospice providers with different agendas and offerings. It's not so easy to be a good consumer when you're in such a vulnerable state. You need to call trusted sources, ask your doctor who they like or consult friends. It's worth taking the time to look into it. At NPHI, we have a phone number that can connect you with a good hospice anywhere in the country.

RJS So many people have a view of hospice as being only end-of-life—as in, you know, "You're going to die immediately." Even Melissa, who served on a hospice board in Ohio—even with all her experience, she also had that notion, and so we only had the benefit of hospice for two weeks. And afterwards, I really regretted it, because they offered so much, beyond anything we could've anticipated.

The thing that held us back was that Melissa didn't want to give up her regular doctors, and that was part of what was required. Once we chose hospice care, we were so happy we did, but isn't it really difficult for families to make that choice of giving up their doctors to opt for hospice?

MM: Yes, it is. As we've said, when you choose hospice, you're choosing to forego curative care. Underlying that idea is, "Maybe this is going to finally catch up to me." And that's the challenge. Often, people struggle with the idea that they're giving up on the person or the patient is giving up. It's one of the most difficult parts for many families.

I have a lot of empathy for folks in that position. If you've had an experience with hospice, you likely would recommend it to everyone. But if you haven't experienced it, it's a scary concept in a culture that doesn't talk about death very well. If I had a nickel for everyone who has told me, "If I had known how wonderful hospice is, I would've called you sooner..."

RJS: Can you share some advice for making the mindset shift to hospice from curative care? It's so difficult to have those conversations.

MM: Whatever else it is, hospice is a symbol of an emerging truth: We are turning toward the idea that we're leaving the world, and we're not going to get better. And what hospice says is, "We're now going to hold you gently (medically, socially, spiritually) in our world." Once that shift begins, it's my experience that often, beautiful things are possible.

RJS: Our relationship with hospice was incredible. Melissa's nurse actually got in bed with her and would just talk with her. It was dynamic and powerful and so kind.

MM: It might be the most intimate thing to be present in those moments. It is remarkable.

I remember another patient, a woman dying of throat cancer, and since she wasn't able to speak, she would write notes. Her husband would say, "We're going to beat this," but we could see that she was near death.

I asked her, "Do you think you're getting better?"

She picked up her pen and wrote, "I know I'm not."

This conversation made it clear to me that she felt alone in this experience, and that needs to change.

I've had patients tell me, "It's so nice that someone will talk to me honestly about where I am." Hospice walks with you in this conversation. In turning toward your leaving, you can find peace, and families can have a sense of real closure.

Family members who've cared for a dying loved one have told me, "This is the hardest *and* the best thing I've ever done." Sometimes, in the curative space—that is, where you are still seeking a cure—there's no room for that conversation.

Eastern religions talk about this. They teach us that as we contemplate our mortality directly, it allows us to live each day as best we can, realizing what's really important. There's a lot of value in conversations about death.

And the conversation is changing. People are becoming more open, but it's still really hard. There's a tension between being optimistic and realistic. We need to hold space for both of those. And hospice can help to do that.

RJS: Speaking of conversation, sometimes it can even be awkward speaking to the doctor. I don't think most doctors are comfortable saying, "You have two weeks to live." Would you agree that even medical professionals have trouble communicating the hard truths that may be unfolding?

MM: I think that's right, but having that conversation should be part of their toolkit.

The truth is so relieving. When you're able to make that turn or that shift in perspective, you're looking for meaning and peace and wrapping up well with loved ones. Sometimes, the doctor's lack of candor denies people the right to "pack their bags" and turn toward leaving.

I once accompanied a rabbi on a visit to a dying man. He was almost in a state of active dying when we arrived, yet sadly, no one in his world had helped him understand. He was still planning to go for one more radiation treatment, and his son was heading back to university. I told the family, "I think he's not going to be with us very long."

RJS: Our hospice team was really in sync. They did communicate clearly, but with a lot of empathy, and it helped me so much. I was in a state of shock, but when I look back on it, they were just so expert at knowing what Melissa needed and even how much time she had left.

Having them there, and having her be at home with me, gave us both a lot of comfort.

MM: Studies have shown, and it makes perfect sense, that people prefer to die at home surrounded by loved ones. Hospice care can be so helpful in accomplishing this.

RJS: Mike, what do you think about newer options to guide people through the dying process? I've heard about "death doulas," for example. I guess they help with various things at the later stage of life? I can see their value, even if some part of me thinks the family should be taking care of it. But maybe we don't want to or don't know how to.

MM: I think it's an important movement. Death doulas, who are called to accompany a dying person as they transition, can provide real value. It's an emerging field. Some hospices are using them, and in terms of being a companion and accompanying a family and patient in this process, I think they can be very helpful. They wear a lot of hats: social and family interaction, legacy projects, meditation and even patient advocacy in some cases.

RJS: My goal with this book and our conversation is to help folks understand that there comes a time when you have to do what's best, and you have to realize a bit sooner that maybe hospice is the best thing. We have to talk about death. We can't let fear or guilt stop us. We need to talk about it sooner rather than later.

MM: Yes, we really do need to encourage these conversations. When it comes to hospice, I'm astounded at how much people don't know about how much good it can do over a longer period of time.

Also, for people who are very ill, at some point in the journey, they intuit or they know, "I might be dying," and I think part of that shift is helping them not feel alone in that realization. There's a way to have "both/and" for a while.

Once, as a chaplain, I visited with a young man dying of ALS. He was in his 30s, and he had a very strong connection to his faith, a sincere confidence in God's plan. He wanted us to pray for God to save him.

We agreed, "Okay, we're going to ask God to save you." After that, I was able to ask him that if for whatever reason that was not God's plan, what is it that he would need to do or say? He thought about it and ended up choosing gifts for his two daughters for their future wedding days. He was able to hold both possibilities in balance and to do beautiful things for his family as a result.

Imagine years after your father's death, on your wedding day, you open a note and a gift chosen by him all those years ago.

In hospice, we don't say there's a right way to do it. It's each person's journey, and we honor that. I've had the experience of walking into a home, the family is in the kitchen and they say, "We know Dad's dying, but don't tell him." Then, we walk into Dad's bedroom, and he says, "Look, I know I'm dying, but don't tell the family." But a spirit of more openness around the subject offers incredible possibility for true connection and resolution.

CHAPTER TAKEAWAYS:

- Educate yourself about the differences and benefits of hospice and palliative care
- Ask your medical team questions early and be your own advocate to help you understand your options
- Be open to honest and clear conversations about end of life, as it is part of the cycle of human experience

"IF I HAD A NICKEL FOR EVERY TIME SOMEONE SAID TO ME, 'HAD I KNOWN HOW WONDERFUL HOSPICE IS, I WOULD'VE CALLED YOU SOONER...'"

—Michael Milward

Chapter 11
GRIEF AND MEMORY

I miss you every day, Melissa.

In this book, I've started most of the letters to you with the words, "Do you remember...?" This time, I want to tell you how much I remember about the way you lived your life.

Beauty seemed to follow you everywhere. You embodied kindness and friendship in all that you did. You met every challenge with humor and grace, and you sure knew how to throw a dinner party.

When you died, even though you had been battling cancer for so long, I was devastated. I knew I couldn't possibly host a celebration of your life immediately, because I wasn't ready. My grief made everything seem impossible. But over the next few months, I became inspired to plan something befitting your style, your personality, your panache.

I hope you got a chance to see all the flowers, the horse and carriage and the special details at the dinners I organized in Ohio, Florida, and Arizona. I wish I could've shown you the shadow boxes I made with little souvenirs of the events for those who couldn't attend.

Most of all, I pray that you heard all the wonderful things your colleagues, friends and family said about you. I pray you felt the love that was present in all those rooms that will live forever in my heart.

Bob

PRACTICAL ADVICE

There is nothing I can tell you about your own grief. It is yours and yours alone, and every one mourns the loss of someone precious in their own way, in their own time.

What I can say is that even though it took me awhile to be able to put together a celebration of life for Melissa, because I was so overwhelmed by my grief, when I was ready, the act of gathering people, choosing details, thinking about words and thoughts to share—it all had such a healing effect on me. With a little bit of time, I was able to accept the outpouring of love and support that was coming my way, and I was able to think about Melissa's life as the beautiful expression of her spirit. That helped me approach her tribute as something more personal and uplifting rather than just a dark and formal funeral.

Below are just a few points that come to mind when I think about how memory and grief are intertwined as we celebrate those we've loved so well.

Take the Time to Celebrate the Life of Your Lost Loved One

In our modern times, there can be a tendency to do things as simply as possible and move on. But mourning in community can be transformational to your own healing. I'd encourage you to read the Help from the Experts section that follows in this chapter, where I talk with two industry experts who share inspiration for how to create a truly personal tribute that reflects the life you're honoring, a tribute that also can help you, your family and community process the grief you're experiencing.

Remember: Grief Is Not a Linear Process and How We Grieve Is Unique to Us

Be gentle with yourself, acknowledge and honor your feelings and give yourself the time you need. One thing that worked well for me after the first few months was creating a policy of saying "yes." Yes to invitations from friends for dinner or brunch. Yes to a family wedding. Yes to starting something new—in my case, studying Spanish, for example. The idea is to try to keep your heart and mind open, even in this difficult time.

When Mourning, Expect the Unexpected

Because grief is not the same for everyone, it can come at us sideways or in forms we don't always anticipate or understand. It can bring fatigue, anger, manic behavior, mood swings and the like. You may feel destructive or out of control. You may be certain that your terrible grief will never pass. Whatever you are feeling, be kind to yourself.

When unexpected feelings or symptoms crop up, get support. Don't isolate yourself, and give yourself plenty of grace. Rest when you can, and try to treat yourself well.

It May Sound Basic, but Reading About Grief Can Be Very Helpful

There are so many thoughtful books, websites and even some new smartphone applications that can guide you through the grieving process, give you more clarity on what you're feeling and suggest thought exercises or other pursuits that may offer comfort and boost your resilience. If you're looking for community, they can help you find that as well. You can also listen to podcasts or join a local support group to help you connect with others who will understand what you're going through.

I've put together a Reading Room section at the end of this book, and I hope you'll take a look. We also post resources on our website, **WeWereBetterTogether.com.**

HELP FROM THE EXPERTS

Although we didn't talk about it a lot (and I wish we had!), I knew Melissa would never have wanted a stodgy, buttoned-up and boring funeral. But the thing is, I was so consumed with grief right after her death that I couldn't even think about it.

To be honest, I was also overwhelmed by how to honor her, and for a time, that was an obstacle to being able to plan and organize. I knew I wanted to do something really special for Melissa, but I had to grant myself the time to be ready to do that. Realizing my own needs and giving myself the space to grieve before creating a formal event was very important for me, and was key to my healing.

In this section, we'll hear again from Father Terry with profound guidance on how to open yourself to your grief in a way that works for you.

Then, we'll speak again with Mike Milward, hospice chaplain and funeral celebrant, along with event expert Karen Bussen, to talk about how our world is changing with regard to celebrating the life of someone special. As preferences shift away from traditional, formal and solemn funeral practices and toward a more personalized approach to remembering a beautiful life, our options are increasing and attitudes are shifting.

At the end of the chapter, Father Terry himself offers a very personal meditation on his own grief experience after the losses of his father and mother.

GRIEVING UNIQUELY: Using Faith, Self- Expression and Connection to Guide Your Journey After Loss with Reverend Terence Keehan (Father Terry)

Robert J. Shearer: I know that many people feel isolated and alone after a loss, as if no one can understand what they're going through. Personally, I wanted to avoid that feeling of isolation as much as possible, so after Melissa's death, I decided to say yes to any invitation if I was available. I am still fairly early in my own grieving process, but I can say that going to a wedding, having dinner with friends, maintaining a determined openness to connection—it has really helped me so far. Do you have any advice for those who are feeling isolated?

Reverend Terence Keehan: First and foremost, we all live, die and grieve uniquely. No one person will experience loss and grief in exactly the same way as another. But since there are commonalities in our human experience, connection can bring comfort along the way. There is magic in confiding in another who can not only sympathize with you, but empathize as well because they have shared a similar pain or loss.

RJS: But what about someone who is really hurting and just says, "Why bother? Others just won't understand?"

RTK: In over 40 years of ministry, I have seen people trapped in the dynamic of, "No one knows what I am going through." Sometimes, it's even said in anger: "You have *no idea* what I am going through."

When it comes to opening up to connection, of course it's true that sharing the details of this challenging end-of-life sequence is unbelievably intimate. It should be held with the most gentle respect and tenderness. But ritual, public prayer, remembrance events and even celebration almost always bring consolation and closure amidst the sorrow of grief.

RJS: Sometimes, it seems that grief is "holding on" to the person you've lost, and it feels like letting go of that grief will be letting go of how much you loved them. Do you have any advice for those struggling with that balance?

RTK: Here's one way of framing it, which many people have told me is helpful to them. The idea was introduced to me by my friend Father Jack Wall, former pastor at Old St. Patrick's Church in Chicago and current President of the Catholic Extension Society. Think of a young child who's learning to ride a bike without training wheels. At first, the parent trots behind the determined youngster, often alternating between holding on to the seat and letting go. If the adult holds on too long or too tightly, the child will never learn to balance by themselves. If there is too much letting go, the child will fall too often and become discouraged. So, we can see in this simple story that there is a fine line between holding on and letting go.

In grief, everything that is human about us wants to hold on to our departed loved one. Our faith, however, tells us to let go: "Let this person go into the loving arms of God."

RJS: I know that in my own experience, I really wanted a way to continue to honor Melissa and also to try to help others going through similar journeys. This book is an expression of that. I've also found a lot of comfort in supporting organizations that were important to her. What are some things that can help to navigate grief in a way that honors the uniqueness of your relationship and still helps you move forward?

RTK: As an extrovert myself, I highly recommend the transactional dynamic of sharing details of this adventure with others. If you can, talk to people about it. You may find energy and clarity as you literally identify your feelings in the process of actually verbalizing them.

That being said, I also realize that we are not all extroverts. Extroverts get energy by sharing. Introverts get energy by going within, so sharing feelings of loss and grief can be that much more difficult for them. It may even add to the pain of a loss. Again, we all grieve as individuals.

In situations such as these, I recommend finding another way to express yourself—something like what you just said, Bob, such as what you've created with this book. It doesn't have to be a formal project or a whole book, but I'd encourage everyone to write and collect their feelings, even if it's just for yourself right now. This may prove cathartic and could quite possibly shift your perspective, bring you to some new understanding or help you record thoughts and emotions that may be difficult to even identify. You can revisit them as a foundation for a future conversation when you're ready. Or you may never share them with anyone, and that's just fine, too.

And remember that you can always speak privately with your faith leader or with a counselor. For those who have more introverted communication styles, this quieter exchange may offer a good solution, especially in the early stages of grief.

And yes, supporting causes or organizations that were important to your loved one is another beautiful way to nurture that connection and keep their memory alive in the spirit of service to others.

CELEBRATING A BEAUTIFUL LIFE, BEAUTIFULLY: Inspiring Ideas to Send Off Loved Ones with Substance and Style from Two End-of-Life Industry Insiders

Michael Milward, CEO, California Hospice Network and strategic advisor, National Partnership for Healthcare and Hospice Innovation

Karen Bussen, Former CEO of the End-of-Life Planning Platform Farewelling and Internationally Known Event Expert

Robert J. Shearer: Mike, how many life tributes have you led as a celebrant, and how have you seen practices change over time?

Michael Milward: Oh my goodness, over 20-some odd years, it's been my privilege to officiate at many beautiful memorial services. All have been very unique, some with just two people at a grave site, others with hundreds of people in a church or more formal setting.

There are so many different ways to celebrate a life, and these events are changing unlike ever before. It used to be that you went to a funeral home or church, and it was a prescribed ritual without much input permitted or required. Now, people can create much more personal celebrations, using non-traditional locations, for example, and take advantage of technology to create visual tributes or bring people together across long distances.

Some of the most significant changes in these newer tributes involve people who describe themselves as "spiritual but not religious." How do we include ritual and spirituality, which are so important to grieving, when a person doesn't fit into a specific faith profile?

If you already have a relationship with a faith leader, a rabbi or a priest, for example, you likely wouldn't seek out a hospice chaplain like me to help with a memorial service. We get called when folks don't have that formal relationship or don't identify as religious. But almost always, they can find a connection to their own spirituality.

More and more, families can find creative ways to celebrate a life, ways that feel like just the right thing for those honoring their special person and like a gift to those attending the event. The community surrounding this person feels *enriched* by attending. They feel, "I am different in leaving than when I walked in." Sometimes, traditional services with more classical language can make it difficult to connect and to experience that transformation, so newer ways of creating rituals around death can open an opportunity to make a shift.

Those attending say, "This was great. I didn't expect this." Of course, people come to an event like this in different ways, with varying relationships to the person who has died. Each of us is engaged in that interior process of remembering, of grieving. If, in the service itself, we can try to speak to that process as well as what really matters in life—if we can begin defining the mystery we call "God" as love—then everyone can relate.

RJS: Yes, I actually experienced this as well at Melissa's memorial service. People loved our celebrant and dozens told me they'd found the whole experience to be refreshing and uplifting.

MM: And spirituality is often welcome even in a non-traditional setting. It may even be needed. As an example, Presbyterian theologian Robert McAfee Brown tells a story about a student who died unexpectedly. His community held a service honoring his life, and it was a very secular, non-traditional group attending. But during the memorial, someone started to sing "Amazing Grace." Brown was astounded at how folks were hungry for that moment of connection.

RJS: I felt it was easier to wait until I could handle the planning. And then, for Melissa, it was only right to honor her with a celebration of life. It was just so much more "her" than doing something very traditional. Her whole life *was* a celebration. The events took place over several days, and holding off for a few months was so much better for me. I could be really present in the moment and connect with others who loved her. Plus, I could add in details that she would've really loved. If I had planned hastily, I couldn't have dealt with all that, and it wouldn't have had the same resonance.

Karen, I know that you started as a wedding and event planner and then became very passionate about helping people celebrate the lives of their loved ones in a more personal, modern way. What inspired this passion?

Karen Bussen: Yes, it started with my sister. I was busy producing weddings and events, and my younger sister was suddenly diagnosed with a rare and aggressive cancer at a late stage. Happily, she came through it and she's fine now, but the experience threw me into a tailspin around mortality, and I became fascinated by how we celebrate a life and why that one essential human experience is so often overlooked and under-personalized.

I decided to shift my design talents in this direction to help people align their celebrations of life with their values, their priorities, even their personalities. It's the most meaningful work I've ever done, and to your point about how people react when they attend one of these non-traditional memorial events, it's just so fulfilling to see with my own eyes the comfort and connection and even relief this approach can bring. And it has nothing to do with budget. It's about designing moments and creating opportunities for people to personally process what is happening.

RJS: Mike, you recently shared with me the script of some remarks you made as a celebrant. It was a life tribute for someone you knew personally. I was struck by how you framed the two parts of the event, to include an "Opening and Centering" and then a "Sending" or letting go. This was something I also tried to do with Melissa's memorial service. Could you speak more about this approach and why it's so powerful?

MM: Yes, both in the Welcome and in the Sending, we say, "We're here to do two things: to honor, remember and celebrate the life of this person, but also, and just as importantly, to release the person to death and to release ourselves to life without them."

Now, when I say "releasing," we're not letting a person go into nothingness. Depending on what is right for each family, we can say they're now held gently in the hand of God, or that we leave them to a place of peace and love where they rest without pain or longing. The point is, we need to name what's happening. That's why we're here: to talk about the completeness of what's going on. Now, we take them from this place for the rest of our lives, and we hold them in our hearts. And we must go forward.

RJS: Karen, once I was ready to plan Melissa's memorial events, for me, it was very important to create something that reflected her—her values, her style, even her design sensibility. When you talk with families who are planning a memorial, how do you help them organize something unique and personal for their loved one?

KB: For me, it's all about the individual we're honoring and the family. I want to know as much as I can. I start with the story of the person. I ask so many questions. I once heard a colleague say something so brilliant and thoughtful, and I now say it, too. In the beginning of our planning, I say, "Let's bring this person into the room."

As we talk, the ideas just start to build. For me, a truly unforgettable tribute is about the feeling, the emotion we evoke. What speaks to who they were in this life? How can we honor them in a way that feels truly authentic? I want people who knew this person to say, "Wow, this was just so her. I felt her presence in every detail." Or, "This is exactly what he would've wanted."

RJS: Since I had a clear vision for Melissa's celebration of life, I wanted to work with someone I could direct. I wanted them to monitor things, to support me in administrative tasks, to coordinate. But I knew what I wanted, I knew what Melissa's family would want.

Because it was a weekend of events, I tried to add in interesting activities—golfing for the guys, a women's luncheon and a trip to a local museum. One night, I had two dinners going on at the same time, because it was really two different crowds and I wanted everyone to feel comfortable.

When it came to the service, we had a great celebrant, but I really wanted to make it unique. Melissa loved carriage rides, so I had a carriage and horse take my sister-in-law and me to the church. We carried Melissa's ashes with us in the carriage. During the service, it was special when good friends did readings. They each brought something of their relationship to Melissa into the moment. Then at the end, Melissa's 11 nieces and nephews and myself, we released 12 doves in front of the church. It really felt like a release.

At the dinners, I asked our friends who are musicians to prepare something special to add a spark to the event. It was wonderful and created that lightness of spirit for a moment that just brought Melissa into the space with us. She would've loved it.

But Mike, do you agree that waiting a bit timewise to plan a memorial can be a good thing?

MM: Yes, it can be very helpful. Of course, in certain religious traditions, funeral or memorial services will take place immediately, or quickly following the death, and the family is well-supported by that faith community in hosting those events. And in my experience, when there is a bit of breathing room and people have a chance to plan, it can really blossom and become something truly unique.

And Bob, listening to how you approached Melissa's memorial is inspirational. And Karen, I so agree with your thought about bringing the person we're honoring into the room. Who were they? As soon as that invitation is offered, people begin to tell stories and share little bits and pieces. Ideas will spring forth as they do.

Two things strike me that are really important. First, if they're able to do it, it can be so helpful for the person who is dying and their family to have a talk about what the dying person would prefer for a service. I've had hospice patients tell me, "I don't want a service, I don't want to be a bother." As we're able to talk this through and they're able to understand how important this event is to their loved ones, there can be a shift. So to the extent that we're able to have that conversation, it can be a true gift.

It's so helpful when we know what our loved one really wants. It can bring great peace to the family. And when you have the opportunity to really honor the individual, that authenticity resonates with the whole community.

RJS: I just wanted to say from experience that if you find yourself without specific instructions, just think of your person and you can figure out what to do. Ask yourself, "What did they love most? What are the adjectives that describe them? How can we bring that all into this moment of celebrating them?"

MM: Well said, and I totally agree.

KB: Exactly. Just find their spirit and follow it. Let it guide you through every decision. We once did a memorial for a young man who died in a car accident. He was an avid fisherman, and he loved tacos and Coca-Cola. We got a special permit from the City of New York to hold the memorial on his favorite stretch of beach. We set up an "altar" right in the sand and asked everyone to bring something to place there in memory of him. They brought fishing lures, photos, notes, little presents.

At the end, we hired a taco truck to park next to the beach so as people left, they gathered and had a bite to eat (and a personalized bottle of Coke that had a printed message: "Have a Coke with Michael"). Everyone I met there said, "Michael would have really loved this."

His mother told me that approaching the memorial in this way totally transformed her experience of grief, that it replaced the tragic circumstances of his death with an empowering moment of really celebrating the amazing person he was and everything he loved in this life.

RJS: A question for both of you. What do you think are some important elements in creating an event to honor your loved one that is personal, but that also offers a healing communal experience for those who are grieving? Mike, do you want to start?

MM: This takes me back to the idea of bringing them into the room. When we personalize a ritual or a celebration, when it is about what we know and love about that person, then it becomes intimate for us and for everyone attending. I'm thinking of my friend Buz, who we memorialized a few weeks ago. He was a guitar teacher. One of his students who attended the service had been taking lessons since age nine, and he played "Into the Mystic" by Van Morrison. This young man didn't say much, just a few words about how important Buz had been in his life. Then he played that beautiful song, and it was so moving.

When we're personal, we make who they were a part of the service. Somehow, that touches the intimacy and mystery within us. When we remember, we "re-member." We put our loved one together again. We make them whole again.

KB: Yes, these are really communal moments where the spirit of that person is almost transmitted or shared within the group, and that's very powerful. There are so many ways to create a moment of communion. It could be as simple as everyone lighting a candle or placing a flower or an object into a "sacred" or special space.

MM: Holding hands or singing as a group or even embracing silence actively—these are also beautiful shared forms of expression to celebrate the person you're honoring.

RJS: And following up on that, Mike, a question about tone. Do you think humor has a place in a celebration of life event? How do you balance the lightness of a funny story or a favorite joke with the sadness and solemnity of a loss?

MM: Humor is such an important part of our lives and how we love each other. In a memorial event setting, I don't think humor ever makes us forget why we're there, and it can provide a moment of relief or even a moment of bonding in the group. People want to laugh, and they want to remember this person in all their humanity. They want to break the tension. The appropriate use of humor is welcome and enjoyed and maybe even important, and it should be used in measure with the person being honored.

RJS: Thank you both for this conversation. I really felt personally that celebrating Melissa's life in a non-traditional way was so appreciated by everyone who knew her, and it has such a profound impact on my own healing. I want to encourage everyone to think about how to make honoring their loved one more special and unique.

Again for both of you, it's true that our society is becoming less religious, but often, there is still a spiritual aspect that is woven into a celebration of life. What are some ways people can add in that aspect of reverence or connection even when their event is not being held in a house of worship?

KB: We worked with a family who had lost a son. None of them were religious, but the mother was a yoga teacher. She didn't have a faith leader to turn to as a celebrant or officiant, and she asked me if she could approach another yoga teacher she knew and liked very much to lead the service.

Although this was a more traditional community, this lovely woman was honored to help with the memorial. She brought with her a few Buddhist elements, like ringing a bell to start the remembrance, and she then folded in everyone else very gently so that they could remember the person being honored in their own special ways. It was so simple and beautiful and authentic, even if it wasn't maybe what you would've expected.

MM: This is a profound question. We may be less traditionally religious, but we all have a sense of spirituality in our lives. What our life means, how we love. There's our interiority that we tap into in these important moments in life. So many families ask me to do services that are spiritual but not religious, but we actually want to tap into our spirituality.

When we come together around love and loss and meaning and existence, we are already in that pool of life energy that we share, and that's a place where everyone can rest without rules and regulations. Music, art, poetry, meaning.

A PERSONAL MEDITATION ON GRIEF AND HOW IT CAN SURPRISE YOU: Reverend Terence Keehan (Father Terry) and His Own Story of Loss

Memory and grief go hand in hand.

If you've lost a loved one, chances are you've already had at least one moment where something unexpected has reminded you of them—a song, a story, or something someone said. Your reaction can be surprisingly intense. Even a small event, encounter or experience may trigger a flood of emotion and grief.

I've lost both my father and my mother, and the reactions I had to seemingly small moments after they passed sometimes really blindsided me.

My dad died in 2006. A love for baseball is a passion we shared. He grew up in Cincinnati, and as a youngster, he and his friends would go to Crosley Field to see his beloved Reds play.

More than once, they watched the Reds against the St. Louis Cardinals, whose best player was left fielder, Joe Medwick. During the game, Medwick would chat with my dad and his friends from the field. He would toss his mitt to them when he and his teammates went into the dugout, waiting to bat. My dad and his buddies would take turns putting on the glove and patting it. When Medwick returned, he'd say, "Okay, give me the glove back," and they would obediently throw it back to him.

About two months after my dad died, I was looking at some

baseball stats, and I discovered that Joe Medwick was 10 times selected as an All-Star. In 1937, he led the league in batting average, home runs and runs batted in, one of only 14 players to do so. In 1968, he was elected to the Baseball Hall of Fame.

This was news to me, and the minute I read it, I grabbed the phone to call my dad. Why hadn't he ever told me how great Medwick was?

Suddenly, I realized that my dad would not answer. He had died, of course, and the reality of his death hit me anew, as if I had completely forgotten it. I became overwhelmed with emotion. Tears came quickly and abundantly. My reaction was a surprise.

Then later, my mom died in 2017. One of my grammar school classmates had brought my parents home after my dad passed away. About six months after Mom died, this classmate, whose name is Cathy, sent me an email to say that someone had commented how beautiful her flowering tree was.

Cathy said she'd told the neighbor, "That's not my tree. It's Pat Keehan's tree."

Again, just out of the blue, I began to cry. This small story of a tree my mom had planted in our yard made me weep, almost uncontrollably.

The point of sharing these two moments is that maybe you've felt something similar. For me, the surprising power of my reactions made me question whether there were unresolved issues with my parents. I spent a lot of time reflecting and realized that the answer was no. It was just love and grief and memory.

Now, I am able to see my tears as an expression of what my parents meant to me, and I am filled with gratitude, even if I still cry whenever I recount these stories.

I hope that you've been able to resolve any issues with your loved ones, but even if not, I encourage you to remain open to unexpected events that may activate your memory and your emotions. Keep reflecting on why they are so powerful, and perhaps you can use them as vehicles to let go of the unresolved as well as cherish the tender.

Do what you can to hold a place for these moments that surprise you in your loss, even if they trigger a response you didn't expect. There is warmth in embracing both the memory and the grief, together.

CHAPTER TAKEAWAYS:

- Grief is a unique and personal journey with no right or wrong
- Consider planning a tribute to your loved one's life as a healing experience, even if you need to wait a bit to do it (remember: there is no rush)
- Even through sadness, direct some of your attention to the beauty of the life your partner lived and what it meant to others
- Take advantage of the wealth of websites, books and support groups that are available (Check out the Reading Room section of this book, or visit us at WeWereBetterTogether.com for more)

"GOODBYES ARE ONLY FOR THOSE WHO LOVE WITH THEIR EYES. BECAUSE FOR THOSE WHO LOVE WITH THEIR HEART AND SOUL, THERE IS NO SUCH THING AS SEPARATION."

—Rumi

Chapter 12
AN OUNCE OF PREVENTION

Melissa,

Strangely, this is a difficult letter to write.

After all, we were kind of the poster couple for a reasonably healthy lifestyle. We were active together, playing tennis and walking everywhere. We worked with a nutritionist to improve our overall eating habits. We took advantage of holistic medicine practitioners and massage. And that was all before your illness!

Some people might look at that and say, "See? Prevention doesn't work." But I'm convinced that that strong foundation we built is what allowed you to continue to thrive for nearly eight years while undergoing numerous rounds of very intense treatments that weren't easy on your body.

Of course, each of us can always do more, but for us, it was always about balance: enjoying life, but in moderation, and using the resources we had to not only improve our well-being but make us feel strong and resilient in our daily lives.

Do I wish there had been a magic vitamin you could've taken to guarantee that cancer wouldn't have chosen you? Yes. Unfortunately, that's not how life works, but I can honestly say we made good choices all along the way, and I know those choices helped us win for as long as we did.

I know you believed that too, and since helping others was always so important to you, I wanted to write about the benefits of preventive health at the end of our book. I hope this chapter will encourage others to take charge of their own health and well-being now, to create a strong foundation for whatever may come, as we did.

Forever yours,

Bob

PRACTICAL ADVICE

I want to start this chapter by acknowledging that if you've lost a loved one, the subject of "prevention" may sting a bit. It may feel that none of it matters now or that you "should have done more." You may feel guilty or like you have no right to take care of yourself now after losing someone you loved so much.

If you're a survivor in remission, you may also be tired of constantly managing your illness, your diet and the like. But I've put this chapter here because I really do believe that preventive practices and small lifestyle changes can help us no matter where we are on our health timeline. I hope you'll read on with an open mind and adopt any of the ideas that feel right for you.

Melissa and I were always keyed into a healthy, active lifestyle years before her illness, but we made sure that it was balanced with how we liked to live and the things that brought us pleasure. We weren't extreme in any way, but we were aware. We were proactive, and it felt good to take charge of our health together, look at resources, make a plan and incorporate small changes into our daily routine.

All that being said, do I ever think back and wish we could've done more? Without a doubt. It's easy to feel that way, but it's not productive.

Does prevention mean that illness will never find you? Of course not. But it can mean that your body and mind are supported by a strong foundation that could help set you up for greater possibilities. And you just might feel better along the way. I really encourage you to think about small adjustments you can make through nutrition, exercise, good sleep practices and other elements, so that's what we'll focus on in this chapter.

Wherever You Are, Start There

Prevention is just a way of thinking about making small or large adjustments to your lifestyle to put your mind and body in a better position to deal with whatever may come. Don't guilt yourself for not having done enough if you already have a diagnosis. Just look at what changes you might want to make now, and make them at a pace you can sustain.

Prevention Requires Support

It can be difficult to make changes in diet, exercise and other daily practices if you don't have anyone in your corner. If your partner is not on board with the modifications you envision, consider enlisting a health coach, a nutritionist or a personal trainer to keep you accountable and to root for your success.

Don't Change Too Much All at Once

Your chances of success diminish if you try to run a marathon before you've even run a mile. Start with the lowest possible expectations. When you meet your goal, you'll reinforce that positive experience, and you can then repeat it several times before advancing to a new goal. Same goes for the number of changes you make at once. Just focus on one thing at a time, and you can gradually add in more new practices to replace those that aren't working for you anymore.

HELP FROM THE EXPERTS

Health and wellness wasn't just something Melissa and I did for ourselves as a couple. We also took steps to create an innovative workplace program of health services, with clinics for our employees at all our locations. We knew that if our colleagues and their families had access to good care without having to miss work just to go to a simple appointment or pick up a prescription, they'd be less stressed and more likely to take good care of themselves.

It was Cheryl Agranovich who helped us establish this program many years ago, and she's been a friend ever since. She's the type of health care professional who not only delivers medical care but who is also a passionate advocate for the community. She's a person who would give you the shirt off her back if she thought it would help you.

She's a big believer in prevention as a tool for better health, and she's an expert in women's health care. I'm so happy she could share some of her advice with us here, and I hope you'll find it helpful as you think about your own health going forward.

AN OUNCE OF PREVENTION: Advice on Taking Charge of Your Well-Being from Registered Nurse, Women's Health Expert and *A Woman's Health Survival Guide* Author Cheryl Agranovich

Robert J. Shearer: As a nurse and a public health expert, I'm interested to know how you found your path to being a speaker and health coach with a focus on women's well-being. Can you talk a bit about your background and what brought you to your current mission of empowering women to build a strong personal health plan even before they have a serious diagnosis?

Cheryl Agranovich: My lens, or my way of looking at health, is multifaceted. I'm a nurse, I'm a survivor of a serious illness, and as a woman, I've experienced the healthcare system on both sides.

In my young life, I was on my own, and I've been financially independent since the age of 17. It was tough, but I knew that education was a way to move forward, even though that had not been a focus in my family. I became the first person in my family to complete college.

At one point, I was actually homeless, and I enrolled in a welfare-to-work program. My counselor said, "You seem smart. Have you thought about a career?"

With his help, I registered at a vocational school to become a nurse's aide. After six weeks of study, I was working and so happy to be able to earn money. I was motivated to continue, and so I then spent a year getting my LPN Licensed Practical Nursing (LPN) degree. Each step increased my confidence, and I went on to earn both an associate's and a bachelor's degree. I also worked throughout my education, and I wasn't homeless anymore.

Then, at 21, I was struggling with an eating disorder that was a result of childhood wounds. I wasn't taking care of myself. It was quite serious. I actually got to a point healthwise where if I didn't change, I would likely die. That was a crucial moment for me.

I decided to live, to take charge of my health. I got into an inpatient program for three months, then followed up with an outpatient program. The experience was a major turning point for me.

I felt like I'd been given a second chance to live. I decided to dedicate myself to help others to be healthier and happier.

Also, in my early work as an ER nurse, I saw patients who honestly should never have needed to be there. If they had just taken more care before—worn that seatbelt, followed their asthma guidelines, gotten that cholesterol under control—they could've avoided a much more serious situation. I wanted to help people understand that.

I spent the next 20 years helping employees through preventive health programs at a number of companies including Mars and Nestle, among others. My goal was always to educate and empower people.

After I sold my most recent company, I decided I'd write a book to help women take better care of themselves and donate all the proceeds to help women pay for their education. If I can help them, it's a great reward for me, as well.

RJS: That's amazing. So before we get into all your advice about health and well-being, do you want to talk a little bit about your friendship with Melissa and the role you played when she got her diagnosis? I mean, you and your husband Vlad have been our friends for nearly 18 years now, and you were two of only a few people who knew that Melissa was ill.

CA: Yes, we really are family now, Bob. I remember the beginning of Melissa's illness like it was yesterday. She and I talked every day several times, and if we were in the same state, we'd usually see each other as often as we could.

So one day, we were all in Florida at the time, and she called me. She said, "Hey, you know I'm having a problem, and I'm concerned. There is some vaginal bleeding."

I asked how long this had been going on. She told me maybe a few weeks or months.

"You're kidding," I said.

She just thought she had a urinary infection or something, but I was immediately worried, although I didn't want Melissa to see how concerned I was. It's just that she had been postmenopausal for a while, and with bleeding over a period of weeks, something seemed off.

I called the hospital immediately because, Bob, you were out of town on business, and we were connected to the concierge service there. We got an appointment for the same day. As we all know, Melissa could be a bit stubborn. She liked to do things her way. But she agreed and she went.

There were a number of different tests, and the next day, the doctor called. She asked Melissa to come in right away.

Melissa called me and said, "The doctor wants to have a discussion with me."

After I offered to drive her, she made a point to say, "Don't say anything to Bob. He has a big week, and I don't want him to worry."

It was a 30-minute drive that felt like hours. I remember Melissa sitting on the exam table, and the doctor came in. She said, "I'm very sorry to share that you have stage four uterine cancer. You need immediate surgery. I've already called the oncologist."

Melissa's face was just not registering. She looked at me blankly and said, "You need to manage this."

I asked her if I should call you, Bob, but she said no, that you were coming home that night.

Right away I called Vlad, and we changed our vacation plans. We contacted University Hospitals Seidman Cancer Center in Cleveland to organize the surgery, because, of course, Ohio is your home base and ours. We'd have to all fly up for that. I knew Melissa was feeling really overwhelmed, so I suggested that before you got home, we would sit down and write a plan of action to share with you. She agreed.

We wrote it all out, booked tickets back to Ohio and got the appointment at UH to see the doctor. Bob, when you walked in from the airport, we were at the dining table. You were instantly organizing. You said, "Okay, we'll take care of this," and that's what you did.

RJS: Yes, it was about two weeks from the day that she went to the doctor until she had the hysterectomy. I remember that first night, coming home and seeing your car was there. I just thought, "Right, we'll handle this like a business problem. We'll figure it out, and we'll do what we need to do."

So now, let's get into some of your best advice. When it comes to preventative health, are there specific guidelines or pillars that we should aim to address?

CA: Absolutely. Taking care of your health doesn't have to be complicated, but it does need to be a priority. Good health doesn't just happen. You can't wave a magic wand and be healthy. It takes a commitment.

When you consider how to approach your own health, think about how you treat your friends. I often say that you should try to care for your body, your mind and your whole self as you would care for others you love. If you can love yourself enough to want to take better care, that's a good first step.

Then also, it is important to reflect on *why* you want to change. Is it for yourself, your family or another reason? I always believe it's best to root your change in what you want for you, but that's not always the case. Whatever motivates and inspires you personally will make a difference.

One thing that's key is that we need to create habits and processes that bring enjoyment to our lives. We often think of change or health-related efforts as not fun, but efforts that feel like a burden often don't last. We need to recognize that change is a process—that you've got to enjoy it, relearn things and build new habits that work for you and that you enjoy.

Other people are also key to your success. We must surround ourselves with people who lift us up and support our goals. This can be tough, because, for example, if you hang out with smokers and you're trying to quit, that's going to be challenging. You have to look clearly at your relationships, reevaluate them and focus on support.

That being said, I believe that each of us is our own health warrior, or the CEO of our health. We're each ultimately responsible for our own well-being. We have to look in the mirror, make our own commitment and take responsibility.

RJS: How do you balance a preventative health plan with still enjoying life and taking into account all the responsibilities and expectations that come with family and work?

CA: Think about the last time you didn't feel great, whether it was a stomach problem, a headache or waking up really tired. How much did that ailment affect your day? Did it impact your work, your relationships, your activities? How often did you think about it? How much attention did you have to give to it? When you're healthier overall, it's easier to live, to find fulfillment and to work more effectively. Studies prove good health makes you more productive toward your goals.

Most importantly, we have to be mindful of the different stages of life and to take our health into account across all those various timeframes. Whether you're in school, starting work, newly married or with a partner, building a family, dealing with an empty nest or even when you're aging, to live better, each of us has to prioritize our health in every phase of our lives.

For example, I made sure that when our kids were growing up, we exercised together. We modeled that behavior to our children so they'd learn that health is important and worth focusing on. In my work, I often take walking meetings with my team to get some exercise while having a productive conversation.

So just to recap, you've got to first make a commitment to your health. You need to make a plan for your well-being and seek support from professionals and those around you. And you need to practice your self-care regularly.

RJS: In your book, I know you talk about creating a "health team." What does that mean in terms of preventive health?

CA: There's so much information out there. It can be overwhelming. It's a great idea to seek out resources in advance and in the absence of a larger issue so that when you're dealing specifically with any health topic, you can get trusted expert advice from someone who already knows you.

RJS: Who are some of the experts that should be on your health team?

CA: First off, everyone should have a primary care physician, a doctor who lives in your community and sees you over time as you pass through different stages of life and health. It's important to build a relationship with your doctor—not just to go when you have an ear infection or to see an ER doctor once, but to get regular care with a physician who will get to know you and whom you can trust. Research shows that we do better when we have a real relationship with our doctors.

For women, a gynecologist is a really important member of the health team, an OB-GYN if you're in your child-bearing years. Through the stages of your life, your gynecologist can educate, advise and guide you, and make sure you're getting the proper screenings, for example.

Next, a dentist. There is research that proves it can be helpful to have someone look in your mouth from time to time, as a variety of health issues may show signs in the teeth, gums, tongue and so on.

Then, checking your eyes regularly and having a baseline to monitor over time is highly recommended, so find yourself a good eye specialist.

A dermatologist may not be on the top of everyone's list, but they should be. Checking your skin at regular intervals and having any suspicious growths looked at is crucial, especially if you have any genetic tendencies toward skin cancer.

I also suggest you identify a pharmacy you like and put their contact info in your phone or address book. Your doctors may need that info, so it's good to have it handy.

Then, there are just a few other recommendations that I think are key to developing the support you need.

Mental health is such an underserved discussion. I think it's essential to find someone to talk to about life challenges. And while I absolutely agree that you should lean on friends and family whom you trust, you should also think about developing a relationship with a therapist over time. This gives you the opportunity to discuss thoughts, feelings, stresses, traumas and challenges in an objective and supportive environment that is just about your well-being.

If resources are available, I highly recommend adding a chiropractor, a dietician or nutritionist and a fitness specialist or personal trainer to your health team.

And then here's one that may seem unusual: If you're someone who has to get blood drawn on a regular basis, finding a phlebotomist you like can be a real plus. Melissa, for example, hated needles. They made her upset, so we found someone who put her at ease and worked quickly and efficiently. It made all the difference.

RJS: What about ideas for people who don't necessarily have a budget for a preventive health team? What can they do to empower themselves and create a solid foundation for good health?

CA: I am so happy you're addressing this. We have to have resources for all. Health is paramount for all human beings. I do have a few to recommend, as I actually used them going through my own journey.

First would be your local health department. You can get flu shots, prenatal visits, diabetes care and other services at low or no cost.

Another great option is United Way 211. They offer support through crises and can provide resources for food and utilities. They're available in most of the US and Canada.

Then there's your local hospital. They'll have preventive care and services for those who can't pay, so don't skip getting seen or having treatment because you think you can't pay.

Planned Parenthood is a solid resource for routine health care at low cost, including sexual health, family planning visits and other services like anemia testing.

And a lesser-known option is that medical schools often provide services for training and research, so you may be able to get eye or dental care or a dermatology exam for little or no cost, for example.

There are also the big associations which can provide help and guidance. The American Heart Association, Red Cross, American Cancer Society and the like.

For fitness, try community centers in your neighborhood. Many offer subsidized, low-cost fitness training workshops and classes or facilities. The YMCA and YWCA are also good for fitness.

RJS: And there's even the idea of going to a massage therapy school for lower-cost massages, which can be so good for your health.

CA: Absolutely, great point.

RJS: Your book explores a number of other important topics that affect health and well-being. What are some of those, and why are they key to prevention?

CA: Well-being involves three main elements: the physical, the emotional and the financial. When we think of health and wellness, we may not instantly associate it with all three of those things, but when one is out of balance, the other two are likely suffering as well.

You may not think that your finances, for example, are connected to your health. But in fact, research shows that they are, and when you think about it, it's clear. If you can't pay for decent food or if you're struggling to keep a roof over your head, you're likely going to have to make other choices that aren't great for your health. It's all interconnected.

For me, the building blocks start with your daily habits like staying hydrated, sustaining your fitness, eating well and getting enough sleep.

And then you build on that with caring for your mental and emotional health, finding your passion in life and even paying attention to your sexual health needs.

Over time, the balance between each will change, but we need an underlying structure to support our commitment to living healthy.

RJS: In my business, when I was dealing with our workforce, I always felt that physical, emotional and financial factors played a critical role in job performance and overall contentment. At our company, we tried to address all three holistically. We offered financial planning for our employees, for example, and we had psychologists on call for our staff.

CA: Yes, I remember that. I witnessed it when working with you on your corporate health programs.

RJS: Sometimes even when we make and follow a plan, disease happens. What advice would you give to someone who is currently battling cancer or another serious illness, whether or not they have a clear preventive plan?

CA: Allow yourself to go through the grieving stages. You can cry, and it's okay to be angry. But at some point, you come up with a plan of attack. When we feel out of control, we can lose our ability to make wise choices. Whatever the issue may be, create a plan. Address what you can control and what you cannot. Focus on what you can control —providers, treatment, your day-to-day routines.

You may not be able to control the fact that you've received a serious diagnosis or even that you've injured yourself in some way. But you can control your reaction, and that can have a huge impact on your recovery. When you take control of what you can impact, it makes your overall experience better.

Then, I'd say it's really important to be your own health warrior. Speaking up and sharing your feelings is crucial, since those around you may not be able to guess and don't want to make a mistake.

Even when it's tough to do so, it's important to help others to support you.

Talk about what you're going through. This allows you to work through the process and the feelings. It's essential to work on the mental health side of things, not just the physical. You have to address both key parts.

Lean in on your faith, meditate or practice yoga. You must connect your mind with your spirit. And I encourage you to seek moments of joy. Bob, I witnessed this when we visited you and Melissa during her illness—you always created moments of joy for her. Melissa used to look at photos on her phone, and then you got her an iPad when her vision began to worsen. She wasn't just sweeping by those pictures. She was genuinely in the moment, you could see it.

When dealing with a serious illness, you need to allow yourself these moments of joy to provide the balance of hormones that can have a healing effect on whatever you're battling.

RJS: For me, those small moments were also joyous. I cherish them even now. One in particular comes to mind—I think it was three weeks before she died. Melissa, at that point, was bedridden and quite fragile. We lived on a golf course, and I remember she said to me, "In a couple of weeks when I'm feeling better, you can go out and play golf, and I'll putt with you."

I knew that the thought of us doing something outdoors together made her happy, even though she couldn't get out of bed. Those little bright spots meant so much.

But just to go back to the idea of support, can you say more about that, even beyond the concept of a health team?

CA: Yes. Outside of the experts, I strongly believe that you need a sort of board of directors for your health—a group of people around you that you can call and who will be there for you. They'll help you stay accountable, and they'll provide support when you need to lean on them. Bob, I know that you were the head of Melissa's board of directors, and she really leaned on you. I like to think that Vlad and I were part of her board, too.

RJS: Oh yes, absolutely, and the folks at UH Connect as well. With us and her doctors, she had all the bases covered, and I know she felt really well-supported.

Switching gears a bit, let's say that, happily, you find out you're in remission or even "cancer-free." How does your health team evolve with you as you navigate your journey?

CA: You still need them, and they'll still follow you as you move into this next phase. But maybe you won't need to lean in as much. And then, taking the idea of paying it forward, if you're fortunate enough to get better, you might think about how you could be a supportive member of another person's team. For someone else who is struggling with a serious illness, having the support of a survivor can bring hope and resilience. I encourage those in remission, who are feeling better or who are cancer-free to give back and be the role model.

RJS: It's true—when you're going through the disease, you feel more comfortable with someone who has been there too. It's kind of like what a good boss or leader does: they understand what you're dealing with from the inside, the trials and tribulations.

Is there anything else you'd like to say about women's preventative health or well-being in general? Your book talks about women's preventive health, but aside from biological details, there's so much men can take away, too.

CA: Well, as I mentioned, I worked in an ER. Anyone who came in for a real emergency surely didn't plan on being there. Statistics show that 14 out of 15 health emergencies are lifestyle related. The 15th relates to accidents, but those also may be lifestyle-related.

My point is simply that when you get your lifestyle aligned with your health, when you have yourself in order, it's both easier to enjoy life and to deal with serious issues when and if they come.

Studies show that 70 percent of how someone feels is related to their lifestyle choices. The other 30 percent is genetics. We each can improve our well-being with some simple changes over time.

It may sound like a cliché, but it's true: Every day is a chance to reset. Instead of worrying about what we messed up on, let's make our next choice a good one.

Come what may, dealing with any issues life may throw at you—whether emotional, physical or even financial—when you approach them from a place of a healthy and balanced foundation, you'll be set up for a better result. Make that commitment, and you won't regret it.

CHAPTER TAKEAWAYS:

- Don't wait to think about preventive care—start now
- Prevention is relevant even when a patient is in remission (and for caregivers and families even after a loss)
- Prioritize creating a supportive healthcare and wellness team not just for moments of crisis but as a foundation of long-term health
- Well-being involves not just physical and mental health, but also financial health
- Start small when making lifestyle changes for your well-being in order to succeed
- You can find resources you need for preventive care, no matter your budget

"HEALTHY HABITS ARE LEARNED IN THE SAME WAY AS UNHEALTHY ONES: THROUGH PRACTICE."

—Dr. Wayne Dyer

AFTERWORD: A PERSONAL UPDATE

As of the initial writing of this book, I'm still fairly early on in my individual process of coping with the grief of losing Melissa. She died in August of 2022, and I spent the rest of that year planning and hosting celebrations of her life in our various communities in Ohio, Arizona and Florida.

I found that having these projects required me to reach out to not just our faith leaders, but also to event specialists, florists, printers and, of course, the people on the guest lists. And that was actually really helpful, because I had something to do that kept me actively remembering Melissa.

With every detail, I thought, "Would she like this? What would best express the fullness of who she was—a stylish, vibrant, funny, elegant, brilliant and kind wife, sister, aunt, business woman and friend?"

Now that most of the tributes are over and the thank you letters have been written, I find myself organizing the next chapter of my life. I sold our large home in Arizona and have moved into something smaller and completely different. I've pushed myself to socialize with friends and go to family weddings and other events to keep me feeling connected.

My thinking is you can choose to be a recluse and withdraw from life, or you can step outside your comfort zone and expand your horizons. I have even started studying Spanish and taking piano lessons, and I've decided to start training with my horses again in preparation for showing them, as I used to do. Of course, moving forward takes time and energy, and you have to give yourself the space to be ready. But a little push can bring good things.

Yes, I sometimes feel lonely. And yes, I still miss my beautiful wife like hell every single day. But I'm moving forward with the help of family and good friends.

One thing I'd like to share is that as a result of my experience with Melissa, I decided to create my own funeral plan, complete with a music playlist and a menu! I'm also simplifying my life just a bit and deciding who will take charge of my affairs, since Melissa and I didn't have children. Doing this is strangely satisfying. I've even written my own obituary, and I don't find that in the least bit morbid.

For people with strong opinions like me, it's a great way to not only take charge, but to alleviate stress and tasks for those who will be kind enough to take care of my funeral arrangements after I'm gone —and this way, I know it will be something that aligns with my values, my faith and my personality.

Other than that, I'm taking it day-by-day. Working on this book has been a gift to me, as it has kept me connected to Melissa's memory every day. It has also given me a sense of purpose, as at its heart, the original idea was simply my effort to serve the community by sharing what Melissa and I experienced and what we learned.

What will life have in store for me next? That is yet to be seen. Will I find love again? Melissa and I used to joke that she'd surely want me to be happy, as long as I suffered a little bit first after she was gone. I surely have suffered—I had the perfect wife and never wanted another, but I am committed to keeping my heart open to whatever may unfold.

Wherever you are on your journey, I send you my thoughts, prayers and wishes, and I thank you for reading and supporting this book. On the next page, I'll close with a poem that means a lot to me. I read it as a part of my eulogy for Melissa.

It was sent to me by Melissa's cousin, Bev Sullivan, and the minute I read it, I felt that it could have been Melissa herself talking. It allows space for both letting go and remembering beautifully.

Robert J. Shearer
Scottsdale, Arizona, 2024

CELEBRATE WITH ME

Is my presence missing? Do you feel a sense of loss?
Then find a quiet place and go inside yourself,
Close your eyes and cup your hands,
Hold my memory with tenderness and love.
Remember the wonder, joy and togetherness we shared.
Feel the energy that we generated.
See us surrounded by golden light.
Hear the rhythm of our voices, a human melody.
Feel us. See us. Hear us.
Embrace us, for I am embracing you.

Now, open your hands and raise them high.
Send my spirit on its way.
Watch me soar! Rejoice as I fly free!

And remember, if you need me;
Close your eyes.
Cup your hands.
Feel the energy.
See the light.
Listen to the music.
Embrace yourself.
Here I am!

—Author unknown

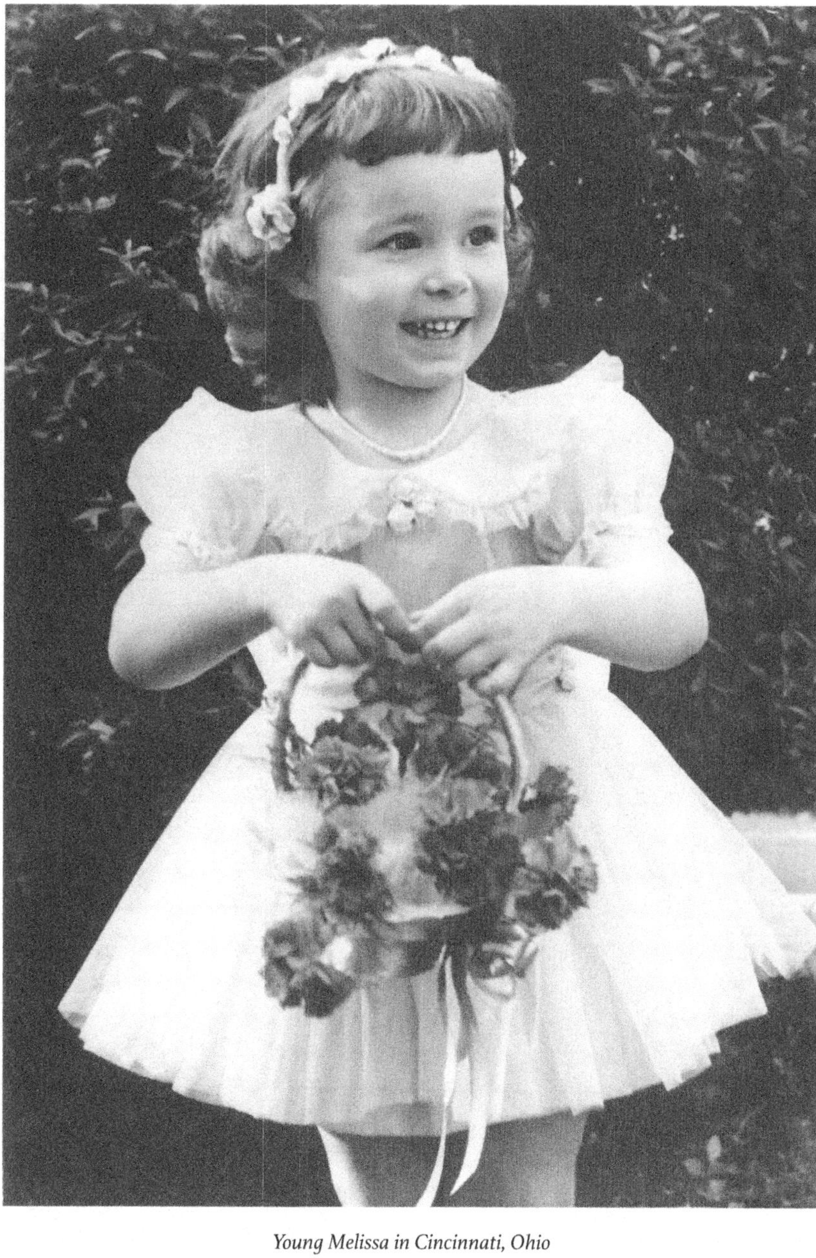

Young Melissa in Cincinnati, Ohio

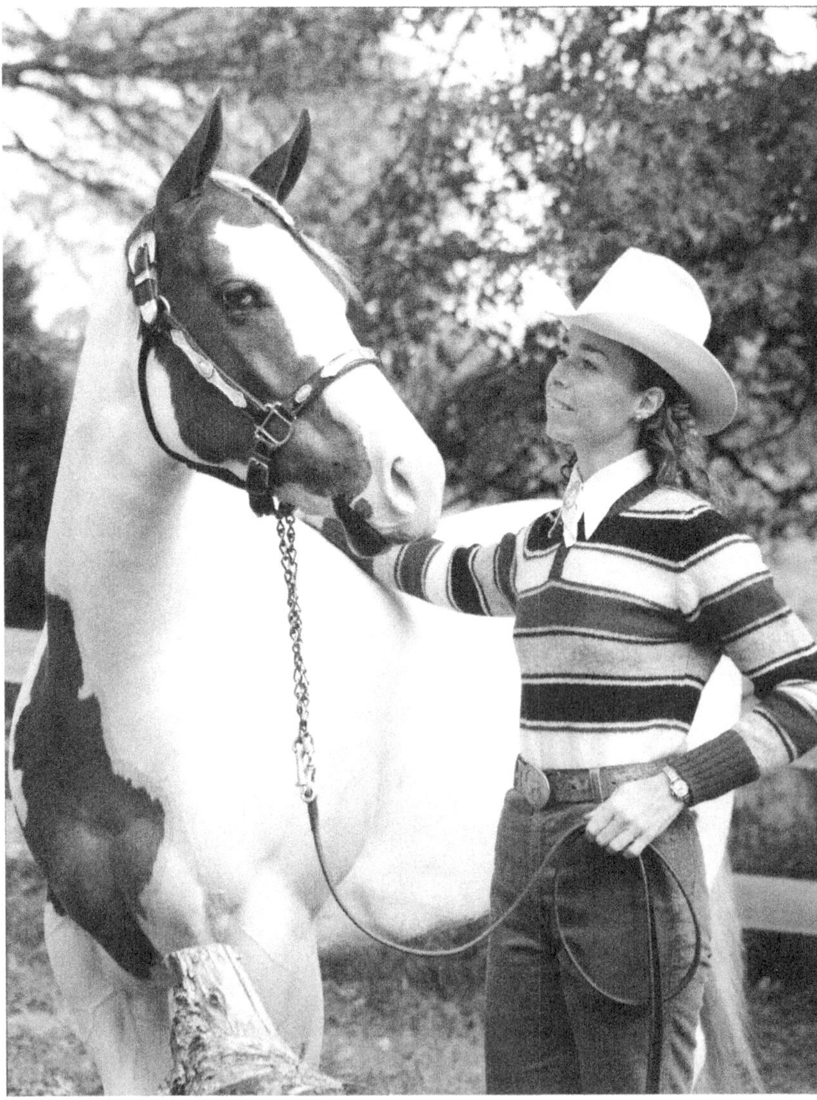

With one of her favorite horses, Tonas Sweet Thing

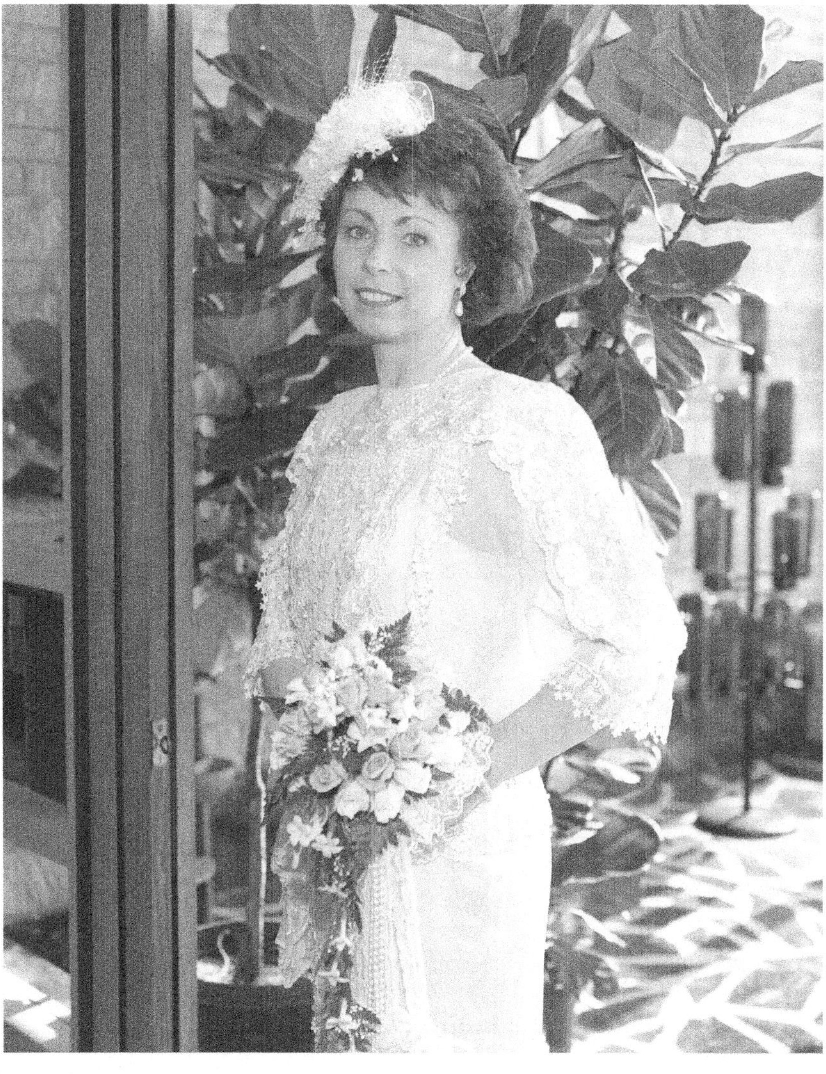

On our wedding day, 1992

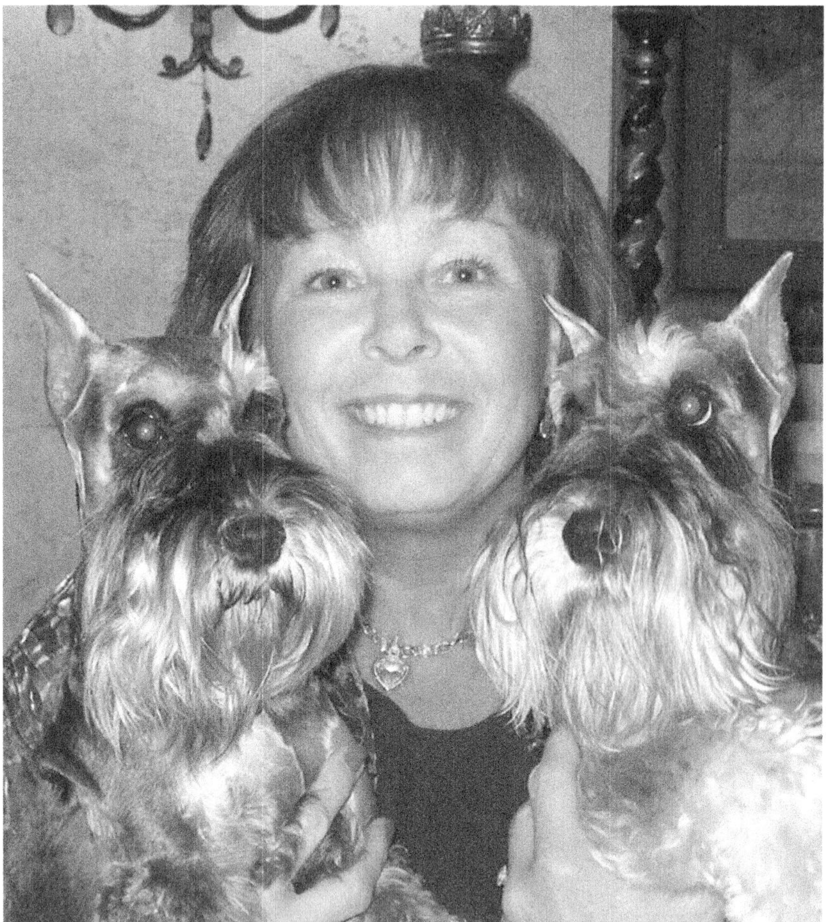

Melissa with two of her beloved dogs

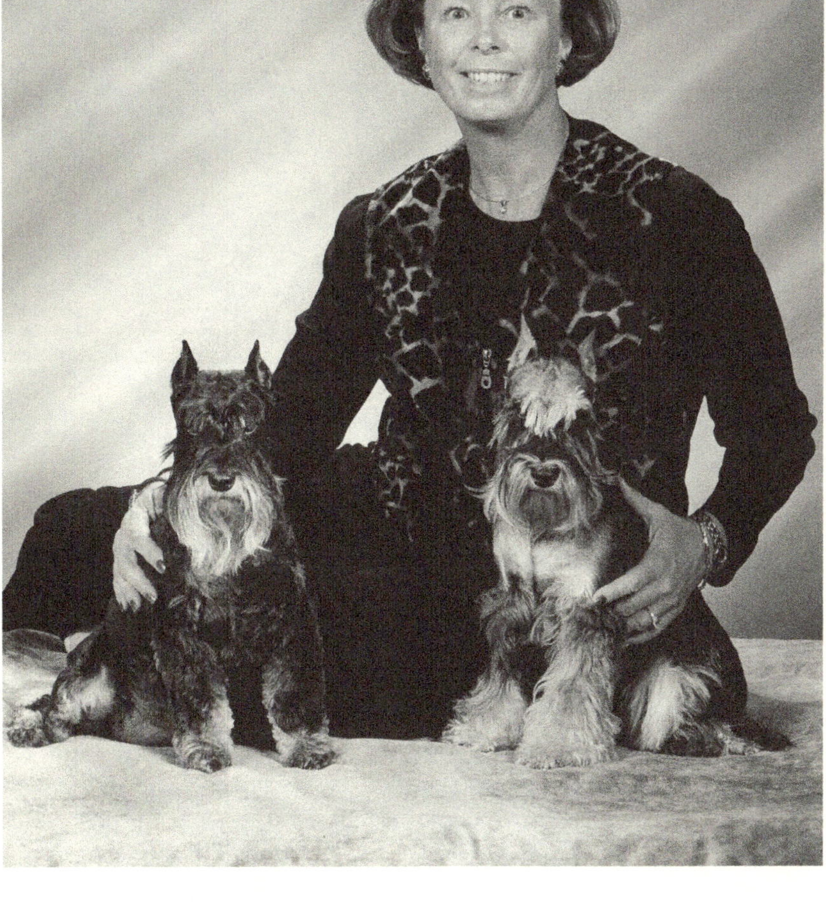

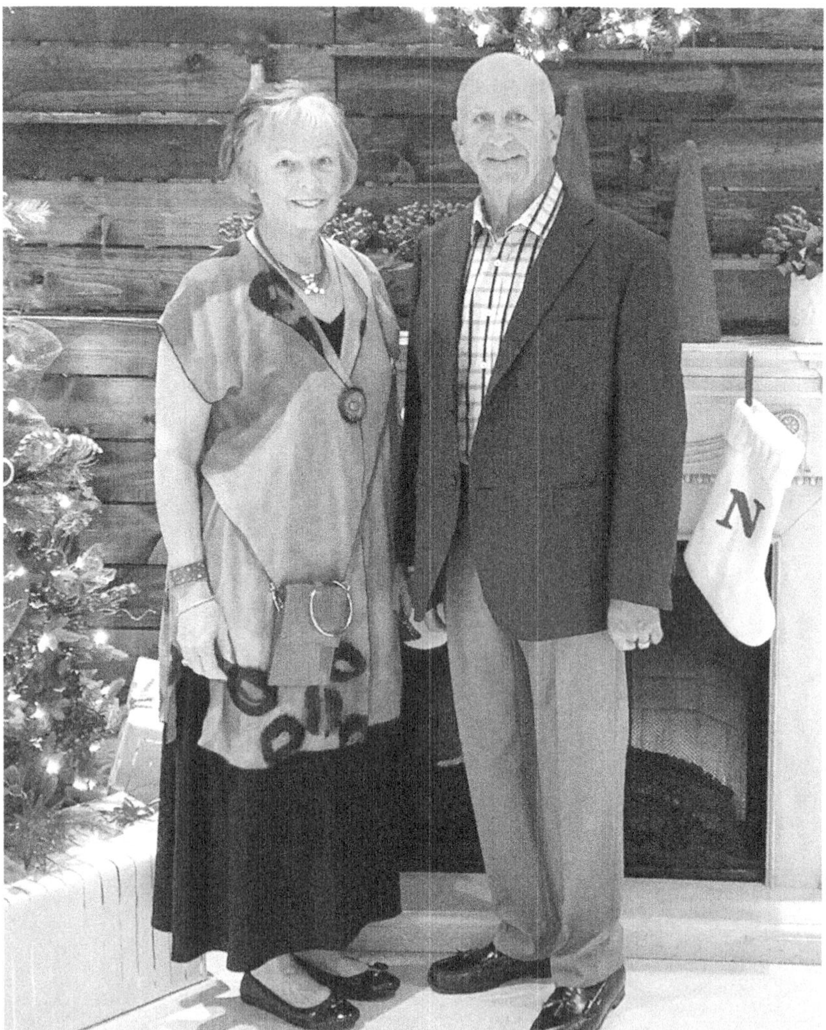

Christmas 2019, Naples, Florida

Scan this QR code for access to more resources, our reading room, or to make a donation to University Hospitals Seidman Cancer Center to help patients and families.

WeWereBetterTogether.com

READING ROOM

Here, we've collected a number of great books that may help you along your journey, broken down by topic. You'll find advice on communicating with your spouse in good times and in bad, tips for focusing on self-care during caregiving and reflections from those who have been where you are now.

The Importance of Communication:

The Five Love Languages, Gary Chapman
The Etiquette of Illness, Susan P. Halpern
The Seven Principles for Making Marriage Work, John Gottman

Personal Cancer Journey:

Calm Your Inflammation, Dr. Brenda Tidwell
Heal Breast Cancer Naturally, Dr. Veronique Desaulniers
The Victoria's Secret Catalog Never Stops Coming, Jennie Nash

End-of-Life Planning and Organization:

A Beginner's Guide to the End, Dr. BJ Miller and Shoshana Berger

Being with a Dying Person:

Advice for Future Corpses and Those Who Love Them, Sallie Tisdale

Self-Care for Caregivers:

We're Stronger Than We Look, Jill Brown
The Conscious Caregiver, Linda Abbit
Caregiver's Survival Guide, Robert N. Yonover and Ellie Crowe
The Soul of Care, Arthur Kleinman

Grief:

The Beauty of What Remains, Rabbi Steve Leder
The Year of Magical Thinking, Joan Didion
What Remains, Carole Radziwill
When Someone Dies: A Children's Mindful How-To Guide on Grief and Loss, Andrea Dorn

Prevention and Well-Being:

A Woman's Health Survival Guide, Cheryl Agranovich
Anticancer Living, Lorenzo Cohen and Alison Jefferies
The First Cell, Azra Raza
Being Mortal, Atul Gawande

Notes

1. BEFORE AND AFTER

1. HSAs are also unique in that they can essentially become triple tax-advantaged retirement accounts beyond being accounts for health savings and investment—after age 65 or if you become disabled, any money you contributed to an HSA that wasn't spent on medical expenses that has been growing tax-free can also be withdrawn tax-free to use on non-medical expenses. This can make HSAs extremely tax-efficient retirement accounts, even better than 401Ks or Roth IRAs, though you have to qualify and follow the rules carefully. (Note: This is not to be construed as financial advice; everyone's situation is different, so please do your own research and consult a financial professional before creating or making changes to any tax-advantaged retirement accounts.)

2. INTO THE WOODS

1. Cuijpers, P., Reijnders, M., & Huibers, M. J. H. (2019). The Role of Common Factors in Psychotherapy Outcomes. *Annual Review of Clinical Psychology*, *15*(1), 207–231. https://doi.org/10.1146/annurev-clinpsy-050718-095424.
2. Lambert, M. J. (1992). Psychotherapy outcome research: Implications for integrative and eclectical therapists. In J. C. Norcross & M. R. Goldfried (Eds.), *Handbook of psychotherapy integration* (pp. 94–129). Basic Books.
3. Fred Hutchinson Cancer Research Center. (2009, November 10). *Men leave: Separation and divorce far more common when the wife is the patient*. ScienceDaily. https://www.sciencedaily.com/releases/2009/11/091110105401.htm.

Acknowledgments

Writing this book has surprised me in so many ways, but none more so than in the overwhelming support I have received during the process.

First off, the generosity of the contributors who donated their time and expertise to help families navigating a serious illness has been unbelievably inspiring. To each and every one of you, my heartfelt thanks for your efforts.

As a first-time author, I have also been grateful for the advice of industry insiders who took the time to point me in the right direction throughout the creative process. Special thanks to Joy Tutela at the David Black Literary Agency and to legal counsel James Gregorio.

The team at Legacy Launch Pad have helped to streamline the project from manuscript to book and audiobook. Thank you!

When I had the idea to create this book, I knew I wanted to work with a writing partner who could help me capture the fullness of all that Melissa and I went through, but also to structure a practical guide that could truly be useful to anyone dealing with a health crisis. I found that partner in Karen Bussen, whom I originally hired to write Melissa's obituary. A few months later, I then enlisted Karen to help me create the eulogy for Melissa's celebration of life, and when it came time to tackle the book project, she was the first call I made.

Over nearly two years, Karen and I have worked together to bring these pages to life. In the process, we've not only made a book that I hope will help a lot of people—we've also built a cherished friendship.

Finally, I want to thank my family and my incredible community of friends in Florida, Ohio and Arizona for lifting me up, taking me into their hearts and gently pulling me forward as I chart this new path. I simply couldn't have done any of this without your love and encouragement.

About the Authors

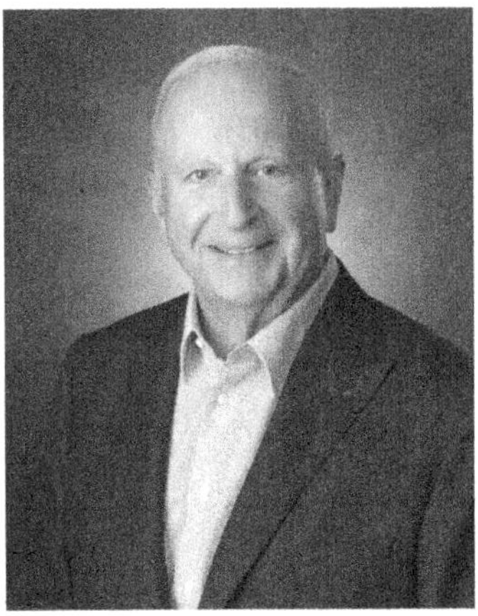

Robert J. Shearer is the Co-founder, former CEO and Chairman of Shearer Foods, a snack food company he built from a single snack distributorship into an award-winning multi-million dollar enterprise.

For 40 years, he ran Shearer Foods, 25 of those with his wife Melissa, who was the company's Vice President of Communications. They loved working together and sold the business in 2012, before Melissa's diagnosis.

Melissa fought cancer bravely for eight years and passed away in August 2022. Bob created this book to honor her and to help others going through a serious health crisis.

Philanthropy and service to the community have always been important to Bob and Melissa, and Bob continues to support numerous charitable causes and organizations.

Bob will donate his proceeds from *We Were Better Together* to University Hospitals Seidman Cancer Center to advance cancer research and to help other families and couples.

Karen Bussen is a Paris-based author and business consultant. An internationally recognized expert in events and hospitality, she is the former owner/founder of Farewelling, an online platform of resources for personalized end-of-life planning.

Made in United States
North Haven, CT
21 July 2024

55198873R00157